Andréa Lima de Sá

Care and attention to Women's Health

Andréa Lima de Sá

Care and attention to Women's Health

An Approach on issues related to Women's health in the areas of Physiotherapy and Physical Education and Psychology

ScienciaScripts

Imprint
Any brand names and product names mentioned in this book are subject to trademark, brand or patent protection and are trademarks or registered trademarks of their respective holders. The use of brand names, product names, common names, trade names, product descriptions etc. even without a particular marking in this work is in no way to be construed to mean that such names may be regarded as unrestricted in respect of trademark and brand protection legislation and could thus be used by anyone.

Cover image: www.ingimage.com

This book is a translation from the original published under ISBN 978-613-9-72355-3.

Publisher:
Sciencia Scripts
is a trademark of
Dodo Books Indian Ocean Ltd. and OmniScriptum S.R.L publishing group

120 High Road, East Finchley, London, N2 9ED, United Kingdom
Str. Armeneasca 28/1, office 1, Chisinau MD-2012, Republic of Moldova, Europe
Printed at: see last page
ISBN: 978-620-6-13228-8

SUMMARY

CHAPTER 1

POSTPARTUM DEPRESSION IN A LITERATURE REVIEW: PREVENTION, RISK FACTORS AND PROTECTIVE FACTORS

ANA PAULA CRISTINA DE OLIVEIRA[1]
CLAUDIANE KÉCIA COSTA DA SILVA[1]
ANDRÉA LIMA DE SÁ[2]

According to Brunner (2011), postpartum depression (PPD) is one of the main complications of the puerperium and represents a public health problem. General estimates on the magnitude of postpartum depression suggest a prevalence between 10% and 15%. However, this seems to be the reality in developed countries, and in less favorable conditions, these numbers can be significantly higher. The consequences of postpartum depression, brings damage not only to the mother, but also to the cognitive and emotional development of their children, as well as the relationship with her husband and family.

Postpartum depression occurs right after childbirth, the symptoms include sadness, mood swings, crying crises and among others. Some mothers experience these symptoms with more intensity, thus developing great psychic suffering. In some cases, the risk factors that predispose to postpartum depression in some women are associated with previous life history, lack of family support, financial problems and domestic violence.

According to Righetti and et al (2003 apud SCHMIDT;

PICCOLOTO E MULLER, 2005), children of mothers with postpartum depression are described as more anxious, are less responsive in interpersonal relationships and their attention is lower, when compared to children of non-depressed mothers. However, postpartum depression is little emphasised by health promotion actions, not giving the necessary importance to the pregnant woman's psychological state, which can trigger postpartum depression in the puerperal period in some women.

According to Zinga (2005 apud ARRAIS; MOURÃO E FRAGALLE, 2014), the method of prevention against postpartum depression is precarious, in which most psychoeducational and hormonal interventions have shown little effect for prevention. However, studies that used interventions with a psychotherapeutic focus, especially in groups, showed favorable results in efforts to prevent postpartum depression.

For Brunner (2011), it is of great importance that health professionals involved in prenatal consultations, even if overwhelmed by the volume of care, are attentive and trained to identify patients at risk, offer support and question aspects related to mental health, opening a space for puerperal women to expose their emotional issues, in order to provide a truly comprehensive care to the health of these women.

Psychological prenatal care is a program to prevent postpartum depression. This work can collaborate with fundamentals of this theme for a better psychological development in the gestational and puerperal period in this phase of life of women and their partners.

Brief psychotherapy with fathers and babies is one of the possible treatments for this situation, since several studies have shown that this form of psychotherapy can have important contributions in the improvement of the maternal mood, in the mother-baby interaction and with the other members of the family (CRAMER E ET AL, 1997).

POSTPARTUM DEPRESSION

According to Rushi et al (2007), depression in Brazil is considered a serious public health problem, affecting the general population. From a medical point of view, depression is a well-defined illness, with symptoms that include changes in appetite, weight, sleep, difficulty concentrating and/or making decisions. It is known that depression does not arise from a single factor but is a multifactorial pathology, in which genetic factors are related.

There are several types of depression, classified as: major depression (where suicidal thoughts are the most serious and the depression is intense and incapacitating), moderate depression (of lesser intensity and may last for a long time) and mild depression (of lesser intensity and where symptoms may persist). In any of the situations, the search for help from a mental health professional is fundamental. Nowadays there is concrete data about the benefits of psychotherapy. It is best to focus on the prevention of depression and the promotion of well-being and happiness (RIVERO, 2009).

Postpartum depression is internationally considered a disorder that affects 10% of women in the puerperium. Minuchin (1982), states that the life cycle is of extreme importance in the puerperium, becoming a special moment. The vital cycle is a process in which biopsychosocial changes and reorganizations occur. It is extremely important that health professionals clarify this phase of the life cycle so that puerperae can readapt to the changes that have occurred. But, unfortunately, in some cases, postpartum depression occurs and makes this special moment a serious risk in this affective bond and in the development of the baby (COOPER and MURRAY, 1995)

Schmidt et al. (2005) state that depression and anxiety disorders in pregnant women usually start between the fourth and eighth week after birth, and may persist for more than one year. The mother may also present mood disorders, including maternity melancholy, known as baby blues or postpartum sadness. In which there is a differentiation between the baby blues (which is the transition of this period and disappears randomly) and postpartum depression (being considered more severe).

The ***baby blues*** is characterized by a short period of volatile emotions, which commonly occurs between the second and the fifth day after delivery, and usually remits spontaneously (O' HARA e ET AL, 1997).

TABLE 1 - Chart adapted from the source: UNGERER, Mariksa Nunes Sanches. **Assessoria papo de gaia**. 2016. Available at: <http://www.papodegaia.com.br/profissionais>. Accessed on: 16 March 2016, showing the difference between baby blues and postpartum depression.

BABY BLUES	POSTPARTUM DEPRESSION
1 Symptoms: Anxiety, crying, sadness and irritability.	1 Symptoms: sleep and eating disorders, sadness, sexual disinterest, among others...
2Duration: appears between the third and fifth day after the birth of the baby and disappears spontaneously in a few days.	2 Duration: it appears in the fourth week after the birth of the child and has an indeterminate duration.
3 Treatment: no medication: only	3Treatment: therapeutic monitoring

occupational therapy, psychological support and physical activities.	and, in some cases, the use of professionally prescribed medication.

Saraiva and Coutinho (2007), state that there are several symptoms of postpartum depression. These include irritability, frequent crying, feelings of helplessness and hopelessness, lack of energy and motivation, sexual disinterest, eating and sleeping changes, feelings of being unable to cope with new situations and psychosomatic complaints.

The risks for maternal depression are related in three categories: the first refers to the quality of interpersonal relationships with the partner; the second relates to pregnancy and childbirth and the occurrence of stressful events and the third refers to socioeconomic adversities. When the mother develops postpartum depression, the child's development may be compromised in difficulties in interpersonal relationships (emotional, cognitive and social) in the future, and may be more anxious and less happy children, presenting fewer smiles, less body interaction and greater eating and sleeping difficulties (READING and REYNOLDS, 2001).

Schmidt et al (2005) mention that the recognition of the symptoms of postpartum depression is important not only for the mother's understanding and treatment, but also to prevent the negative effects on the relationship between mother and baby, and on the child's learning and social and emotional development. Depression during the puerperal period can hinder the mother's adequate stimulation of the baby, which can lead to malnutrition of the child, maltreatment or even infanticide (BAPTISTA e ET AL, 1999).

From the perspective of Health Psychology, it is considered that health/education professionals who are involved in work with pregnant women play an important role in this recognition, diagnosing and referring families for psychological care, and with this work they may assist in healthy child development (SCHMIDT e ET AL, 2005).

The multiprofessional action with pregnant women should encompass the interaction of many factors. Among them, the personal history, the gynaecological and obstetric history, the historical moment of pregnancy, the social, cultural and economic characteristics in force and the quality of care. This should be integral and capable of providing the woman and the child with a satisfactory period of well-being, aiming at strengthening the mother-fetus bond (Falcone et al., 2005).

The puerperium is a special moment in the life cycle, when great changes take place and therefore it is subject to crises in the reorganization of the new roles to be played in the family. Many times these readjustments become difficult and can appear related to a depressive process in the mother, which can have repercussions on the whole family (MINUCHIN, 1982).

When maternal sadness persists or intensifies, the patient may be developing depression, in which the clinical diagnostic criteria are the same as those of the Diagnostic and Statistical Manual of Mental Disorders (DSM-IV) for major depression, which considers the duration of the event in at least 2 weeks, with at least five of the following symptoms: depressed mood, anhedonia, significant changes in weight or appetite, insomnia or hypersomnia, agitation or psychomotor retardation, fatigue, feelings of worthlessness or guilt, diminished ability to think, to concentrate, indecision, recurrent thoughts of death. The onset of symptoms in the first four weeks is only specifying (SUSMAN, 1996).

Depression can be neglected by the depressed mother herself, her partner and even family members, who believe that the symptoms presented by the mother are due to the natural exhaustion and weariness of the puerperium process, caused by the accumulation of domestic chores and the care provided to the baby (CRUZ e ET AL, 2005).

People with marital conflict have from 4 to 25 more risk of developing depression than people who do not report marital dissatisfaction, both in clinical and non-clinical samples (DESSAULLES e ET AL 2003). According to Cruz and et al (2005), the higher the perception of social support from the husband or partner, the lower the prevalence of maternal depression. This means that the partner's support may have a protective effect on the mother's mental health after the birth of the baby.

Meighan et al (1999), the occurrence of maternal depression during this phase can have a devastating effect on both the mother, the child and the rest of the family. Living with a depressed woman on a daily basis may trigger psychiatric illnesses in men, such as anxiety disorders and episodes of generalised depression.

According to Arrais e et al (2014), the psychological prenatal care (PNP), a differentiated approach from the courses for pregnant women, is a modality of care rarely found in obstetric services. Because it is a new perinatal care, directed towards greater humanisation of the gestational process, childbirth and the constitution of parenthood.

The main objective of the psychological intervention is to offer a qualified and differentiated listening about the pregnancy process, as well as to be able to provide a space in which the mother expresses her fears and anxieties, collaborating in the exchange of experiences, discoveries and information, with an extension to the family, especially the spouse and grandmothers, in view of their presence in the pregnancy and puerperium and sharing of parenthood (ARRAIS e ET AL, 2014).

The objective of the research was to identify in a literature review the knowledge produced on the topic, investigating the possible causes of postpartum depression and the identification of the postpartum prevention mode in public health. Within this perspective the best way to prevent postpartum depression is to avoid such effects, and social support becomes one of the factors of prevention (KLAUS E ET AL, 2000).

METHODOLOGY AND PROCEDURES

The survey of this study was based on a narrative review of publications from national and international journals. The studies were initially analysed and reviewed through their titles, abstracts and results. Ninety (90) articles were selected for evaluation of their entirety, and at this stage, three (3) articles were excluded for presenting duplicity and not being relevant to the research.

An initial search was conducted with the objective of identifying relevant articles for the database, that is, other important references not captured by the initial search. All search processes took place in the electronic database, selection of studies, reading of articles, thus aiming at greater reliability of the study.

Identification and selection criteria

The search for articles was conducted in the database, Scientific Electronic Library Online (SCIELO), GOOGLE ACADÊMICO, Electronic Periodicals in Psychology (PEPSIC). The articles were obtained through the following key words: "postpartum depression, risk factors, epistemology, prevention and treatment". The search for references was limited to articles written in Portuguese and English published between the years 2006 and 2016.

Assessing the validity of the study

The articles identified in the search strategy had their content assessed by two researchers in independent and subsequently dependent forms for relevance selection. Through a preliminary reading of the abstracts of 90 articles in order to search for the methodological quality of the selected articles, they were analysed and classified.

RESULTS AND DISCUSSION

According to Ruschi et al (2007), Brazil is a country in which a significant number of women are illiterate or have difficulties in reading and understanding texts. It is noteworthy that these women may even be more likely to present the disease because they do not have the means to help them seek information easily.

Schooling contributes to the onset of postpartum depression. It is verified that the number of women with postpartum depression is significantly higher in women who have incomplete high school education when compared to women who have complete high school education.

The schooling of these women is a risk factor for the development of postpartum depression since most of these mothers are adolescents, many are primiparous and lack adequate information about the pregnancy process and the basic care of the baby. Besides that, women without schooling often submit themselves to low quality jobs and with a lot of physical effort such as, for example, day labourers, cleaners, and freelancers to help the family income. Thus, some women cannot afford a health insurance plan and end up depending on the SUS (Single Health System).

Os resultados revelam que há uma associação de intensidade com sintomatologia depressiva materna, em que descreve a medida que aumenta o grau inferior de escolaridade apresentam um nível maior de sintomatologia. Mas, quando os níveis mais elevados de escolaridade apresentam valores mais baixos de sintomatologia, em que reduzirá os casos de DPP.

Martins and Pires (2008) state that a woman with postpartum depression is a woman who is unavailable to her partner and her baby. In this sense, in an attempt to soften the effects, some studies point out the paternal role during this period. The father appears in this context as a fundamental subject, with a double role, since the well-being of the companion and the baby's development seems to depend on him.

When the first baby is born, there is a decline in the quality of the marital relationship, but the father's involvement and support ensures a significant protective effect against this marital dissatisfaction and similarly against the mother's stress during this period (FELDMAN, 2000).

It can be noted as a characteristic for the triggering of post-partum depression a not stable conjugal relationship. However, when this relationship of the couple is stable, it predominates as a protective factor against PPD. The stable marital situation, predominates the stable relationship between the couple, that is, when there is good affection between the couple and the bond is well established.

According to the data pointed out, the quality of the interpersonal relationships of the mother, in particular with her partner collaborates in a way to prevent postpartum depression, because the lack of conjugal support becomes a risk event within this factor. All this occurs also because of the difficulty in organizing the couple's time, in communication, in the quality of the marital and sexual relationship.

For Garcia and Tassara (2003), the lack of time for the man and the woman due to great work demands is one of the great problems for the conjugal situation.

It is extremely important that the partner is instructed in order to transmit security to the woman, showing that she is not alone, that she will get better and mainly that she is playing her maternal role well (BARNES, 2006). When the father is dedicated he mediates the mother's interaction with the baby, having a direct influence on the child's development and exercising a protective function at this moment (BRAZELTON et al., 1992).

Hops, e et al (1987), state that when there is a good relationship between the couple, fathers in families in which the mother is depressed, have a greater involvement with the children, than the mothers themselves. By adapting a model of sensitive and adequate interaction to the needs of the baby, parents partially compensate for the negative or insufficiently good interaction of the mother-baby relationship.

According to Brunner (2011), lifestyle habits such as alcohol misuse, smoking and illicit drugs by women were associated with significantly higher prevalence of PPD. In relation to the misuse of alcohol by the partner, it is clear that this condition affects the couple's relationship, affecting the support that this partner can offer the woman and leading to the development of postpartum depression.

Alcoholism is seen as one of the most pronounced risk factors in women's partners. It is important to emphasize that this data only prevails when there is a history of alcoholism. When there is no history of alcoholism, this factor becomes similar in both parties (women and men).

Risks are understood as the factors or negative events that are configured as predictors, increasing the degree of tension, influencing individual or environmental responses that increase the vulnerability of the development of a healthy life of the individual, affecting aspects of physical, social and emotional order (MORAES e ET AL, 2006).

The risk factors that most influence postpartum depression in puerperae are: primipara being the index factor that predominates the first place, in second place the unplanned pregnancy and in third place is similar between impoverished support network and post traumatic or unsatisfactory delivery.

These risk factors make it clear that if there is no multidisciplinary intervention as soon as these symptoms appear or are detected, the degree will only increase more and more.

The protective factors are conditions associated with influences that can promote a psychological well-being of the puerpera in order to provide a better response against certain risk events. (ARRAIS e ET AL, 2014). The protective factors that help prevent postpartum depression are: family support, favorable socioeconomic situation, the desired pregnancy, satisfactory delivery and others. At this time, the physical and psychological preparation also helps as a support for the changes that come with motherhood, such as the application of exercises (yoga, hydrogymnastics during pregnancy with professional monitoring, Pilates, hiking and others). As for the psychological preparation, one can highlight specialized preparation courses for baby care.

> In this sense, the protective factors of postpartum depression are preventive measures or situations already established that influence as protection against emotional problems during pregnancy and postpartum period(GOLSE, 2002).

Postpartum depression is a serious public health problem. Within this context, the training of healthcare professionals for the early recognition of postpartum depression is of utmost importance. Teamwork is essential for the protection of women regarding emotional problems and other issues related to the pregnancy cycle. Thus, courses are offered for pregnant women and assistance and guidance programs during prenatal psychology that aim to provide support to women with PPD (ROSENBERG, 2007).

The results of the present study reveal very clearly the influence of the aspects related to the triggering of post-partum depression and prevention as a protective factor. In general, it is perceived that postpartum depression is very much associated with schooling, conjugality and alcoholism as well as other risk factors mentioned in the images above.

CONCLUSION

It is known that due to the lack of prevention of postpartum depression in the prenatal period along with the lack of professional guidance, some mothers in the puerperal period undergo treatment and the cases become increasingly frequent. Thus, this article contributes to the discussion on the subject by highlighting the importance of psychological prenatal care as a way of maintaining the psychological well-being of the mother and defending the healthy development of the children born.

Health professionals at the time of psychological prenatal care should initially look towards prevention. It is known that little emphasis is placed on health promotion and that there is no necessary attention to the psychological state of the pregnant woman at this time.

Currently, postpartum depression becomes difficult and treatment due to its multifactorial character and it is of utmost importance, an early and effective treatment, because the damage in the mother-baby relationship and in the family structure can be irreparable.

It is understood that the problems of women with postpartum depression should be welcomed in order to understand their complaints, their suffering and their difficulties, perceiving the possible causes to better understand and try to alleviate the problems and symptoms that are often interfering with their social life. They should also seek new measures in the exercise of their professionalism when they notice that an approach is not being well absorbed.

BIBLIOGRAPHIC REFERENCES

ALIANE, Poliana Patrício. MAMEDE, Marli Vilela. FURTADO, Erikson Felipe. **Systematic review on the risk factors associated to postpartum depression.** Vol. 5, N° 2, Juiz de Fora, 2001.

AGRA, Sandra Cristina Mendes. **Factores de vida e a intensidade da sintomatologia depressiva no pós-parto.** Instituto Superior Miguel Torga. Coimbra, 2009.

AMORIM, Sonía Patrícia Torres. **Tristeza pós parto: importância do diagnostico precoce.** Fernando Pessoa University. Ponte Lima, 2010.

ARRAIS, Alessandra da Rocha. MOURÃO, Mariana Alves. FRAGALLE, Bárbara. **O pré- natal psicológico**

como programa de prevenção à depressão pós-parto. Vol. 23. São Paulo, 2014.

BAPTISTA, Makilim Nunes. BAPTISTA, Adriana Said Daher. OLIVEIRA, Maria das Graças de. **Depression and gender: why do women depress more than men?** Vol. 7. São Paulo,1999.

BAPTISTA, Makilim Nunes. BAPTISTA, Adriana Said Daher. TORRES, Erika Cristina Rodrigues. **Association between social support, depression and anxiety in pregnant women.** Revista de psicologia da Vetor, vol. 7, São Paulo, 2006.

BARNES, D. **Postpartum depression: its impact on couples and marital satisfaction.**Journal of Systemic Therapies.25 (3).2006.

BELSKY, J., GILSTRAP, B & ROVINE, M.**The Pennsylvania infant and family development project, I: Stability and change in mother-infant and infant interaction in a family setting at one, three and nine months.**ChildDevelopment. 1984.

BRAZELTON, T. B. & CRAMER, B. G. **As primeiras relações.** São Paulo: Martins Fontes, 1992.

BRUNNER, Maria Alice Cortez. **Prevalence of postpartum depression among women assisted in the postnatal clinic of the Fernandes Figueira Institute - Fiocruz**. Rio de Janeiro, 2011.

CANTILINO, Amaury. ZAMBALDI, Carla Fonseca. SOUGEY, Everton Botelho. JUNIOR, Joel Rennó. **Psychiatric disorders in the postpartum period.** Universidade Federal de Pernambuco. University of São Paulo Medical School, 2009.

CANTILINO, Amaury. ZAMBALDI, Carla Fonseca. SOUGEY, Everton Botelho. **Obsessive-compulsive symptoms in postpartum depression: case report.** Psychiatric Journal. Rio grande do Sul, 2008.

CARVALHO, P. **Pregnancy and Psychopathological Risk**. Master's Thesis in Clinical Psychology. Department of Psychology and Education - University of Beira Interior, 2006.

CORREIA, Karyne Mariano Lira. BORLOTI, Elizeu. **Women and depression: a behavioural-contextual analysis.** Federal University of Espírito Santo, 2011.

COOPER, P. J. & MURRAY, L. **Course and recurrence of postnatal depression: Evidence for the specificity of the diagnostic concept.** British Jounal of psychiatry. 166. 191-195, 1995.

COUTINHO, Maria da Penha de Lima. SARAIVA, Evelyn Rúbia de Albuquerque. **Postpartum Depression: theoretical considerations.** João Pessoa, 2008.

CRAMER, B. G. **Psychodynamicperspectivesonthetreatmentofpostpartumdepression.**In: L. Murray & P. J. Cooper (Eds), Postpartumdepressionandchilddevelopment. New York, NY: The Guilford Press. 1997.

CRUZ, ElianeBezerra da Silva.SIMÕES, Gláucia Lucena. CURY-FAISAL, Alexandre. **Screening for postpartum depression in women assisted by the family health program.** RevBrasGinecolObstet, 2005.

FALCONE, Vanda Mafra. MÃDER, Custódia Virginia De Nóbrega. NASCIMENTO, Christianne Freitas Lima. SANTOS, Joacira Mota Matos. NÓBREGA, Fernando José de. **Atuação multiprofissional e a saúde mental de gestantes.** Rev. Saúde Pública 39 (4). São Paulo, 2005.

FELDMAN, R. **Parents convergence on sharing and marital sactisfaction, father involvement, and parent-child-relationship at the transition to parenthood.**Infant Mental Health Journal. 2000.

FONSECA, Vera Regina. SILVA, Gabriela Andrade da. OTTA, Emma. **Relationship between postpartum depression and maternal emotional availability.** Cad. Saúde pública, Rio de Janeiro, 2010.

FIGUEIREDO, Bárbara. COSTA, Raquel. PACHECO, Alexandra. **Prevalence and predictors of depressive symptomatology after childbirth.** Porto Portugual, 2007.

FRIZZZO, Giana Bitencourt. **Contribuições da psicoterapia breve pais-bebê para a conjugalidade e para a parentalidade em contexto de depressão pós-parto.** Porto Alegre, 2008.

FRIZZZO, Giana Bitencourt. PRADO, Luiz Carlos. LINARES, Juan Luis. PICCININI, Cesar Augusto. **Postpartum Depression: Evidence from two Clinical Cases.** Federal University of Rio Grande do Sul. Porto Alegre, 2008.

SOURCE, Rui. **Depressive disorder/depression disorder.** 2010. Available at: <http://www.vladman.net/depressao.php>. Accessed on: 18 Mar. 2016.

GARCIA, M. L. T. & TASSARA, E. T. O. **Problemas no casamento: uma análise qualitativa.** Estudos de Psicologia-Natal, 8 (1), 127-133, 2003.

GOLSE, B. **Depressão do bebê, depressão da mãe: conceito de psiquiatria perinatal.**p. 232- 248. Brasília, 2002.

HOPS, H., BIGLAN, A., SHERMAN, L., ARTHUR, J., FRIEDMAN, L. & OSTEEN, V. **Home observations of family interactions of depressed women.**JournalofGonsultingandClinicalPsychology. 1987.

KLAUS, M. H., KENNEL, J. H. & KLAUS, P. **Vínculo: construindo as bases para um apego seguro e para a independência.** Porto Alegre: Artes Médicas, 2000.

IACONELLI, Vera. **Postpartum depression, postpartum psychosis and maternal sadness.** Revista Pediatria Moderna, vol. 41, 2005.

JUNIOR, Hudson Pires de Oliveira Santos. SILVEIRA, Maria de Fátima de Araujo. GUALDA, Dulce Maria Rosa. **Postpartum Depression: a latent problem.** Porto Alegre RS, 2009.

KERBER, Suzi Roseli. FALCETO, Olga Garcia. FERNANDES, Carmem Luiza C. **Conjugal problems and other factors associated with postpartum psychiatric disorders.** Porto Alegre, 2011.

LOBATO, Gustavo. MORAES, Claudia L. REICHENHEIM, Michael E. **Magnitude of postpartum depression in Brazil: a systematic review.** Rev. Bras. Matern.Child Health. Recife, 2011.

MATTAR, Rosiane. SILVA, Eliza YoshikoKochi. CAMANO, Luiz. ABRAHÃO, Anelise Riedel. COLÁS, Osmar Ribeiro. NETO, Jorge Andalaft. LIPPI, Umberto Gazi. **Domestic violence as a risk indicator in screening for postpartum depression.** Ver. bras. Ginecol. Obstet. São Paulo, 2007.

MARTINS, Debora. PIRES, Antonio Pazo. **The parenting behaviour of companions of women with postpartum depression.** Lisboa. 2008.

MINUCHIN, S. **Familias: Funcionamento e tratamento** (J. A. Cunha, Trans.) Porto Alegre: Artes médicas, 1982.

MORAES, Inácia Gomes da Silva. PINHEIRO, Ribeiro Tavares. SILVA, Ricardo Azevedo da. HORTA, Bernardo Lessa. SOUSA, Paulo Luis Rosa. FARIA, Augusto Duarte. **Prevalence of postpartum depression and associated factors.** Pelotas RS, 2006.

NÓBREGA, Fernando José de. **Atuação multiprofissional e a saúde mental de gestantes.** Centro de promoção e atenção a saúde. Teaching and Research Institute. Hospital Albert Einstein. São Paulo, 2005.

NONACS, R. & COHEN, L. S. **PostpartumPsychiatricSyndromes.**In: B. J. Sadock& V. Sadock (Eds). Kaplan & Sadock's Comprehensive Textbook of Psychiatry (8° ed.). Lippincott Williams & Wilkins, 2005.

NUNES, Maria Ângela Fávero. SANTOS, Manoel Antônio dos. **Depressão e qualidade de vida em mães de crianças com transtornos invasivos do desenvolvimento.** São Paulo, 2010.

O,HARA, F. **The nature of postpartum depression.** In Cooper, P. & Murray, L. Postpartum depression and child development (pp. 3-31). New York: Guilford, 1997.

PROCHNOW, Laura Pithan. LOPES, Rita de Cássia Sobreira. **A relação da mãe em situação de depressão com suas figuras femininas de apoio.** Rio Grande doSul, 2007.

READING, R. & REYNOLDS S. **Debt, social disadvantage and maternal depression.**Social Science Medicine, 53. 2001.

RIGHETTI, V. M., BOUSQUET, A. & MANZANO, J. **Impact of postpartum depressive syntoms on mother and her 18-monht-old- infant.**EuropeanChildandadolescentpsychiatry. 2003.

RIVERO, Catarina. **Depression: A challenge to emotions.** Lisbon, 2009.

ROSENBERG, J. L. **Transtornos psíquicos da puerperalidade.** In: BORBOLETTI, F. F. et al. Psicologia na prática obstétrica: abordagem interdisciplinar. Barueri: Manole, 2007.

RUSCHI, Gustavo Enrico Cabral. SUN, SueYazaki. MATTAR, Roseane. FILHO, Antônio Chambô. ZANDONADE, Eliana. LIMA, Valmir José De. **Epidemiological aspects of postpartum depression in a Brazilian sample.** São Paulo, 2007.

SARAIVA, Evelyn Rubia de Albuquerque. COUTINHO, Maria da Penha de Lima. **A estrutura das**

representações sociais de mães puerpéras acerca da depressão pós-parto. Vol.12. Paraíba, 2007.

SCHMIDT, EluisaBordin. PICCOLOTO, Neri Maurício. MULLER, Marisa Campio. **Postpartum depression: risk factors and repercussions on child development.** Universidade São Francisco. São Paulo, 2005.

SILVA, Francisca Claudia Sousa da. ARAUJO, Thiago Moura de. ARAUJO, Márcio Flávio Moura de. CARVALHO, Carolina Maria de Lima. CAETANO, JoselanyÁfio.
Depressão pós-parto em puérperas: conhecendo interações entre mãe, filho e família. Fortaleza CE, 2010.

SILVA, MaiaraKohlrausch Pires da. ROCHA, Claudine Rodembusch. **O reflexo da violência praticada pelas mães no período gestacional contra seus filhos.**2014.

SUSMAN, JL. **Postpartum depressive disorders.** J FamPract. 1996.

UNGERER, MariksaNunesSanches. **Assessoria papo de gaia:** advice to pregnant women and family. 2016. Available at: <http://www.papodegaia.com.br/profissionais>. Accessed on: 16 mar. 2016.

ZINGA, D, et al. **PPD: we know the risks, but can we prevent it? Revista Brasileira de psiquiatria.**vol. 27. São Paulo, 2005.

CHAPTER 2

THE BENEFITS OF PHYSICAL ACTIVITY AND EXERCISE ON THE QUALITY OF LIFE OF PEOPLE WITH DEPRESSION

FRANCIS MARY DO NASCIMENTO[1]
ANDRÉA LIMA DE SÁ[2]

According to data from the World Health Organization (WHO), depression affected more than 350 million people worldwide in 2015, 5 million of them in Brazil. The data acquired show that by 2020 depression will be the key disabling disease worldwide. Depression has been identified as one of the ten leading causes of disability in the world, limiting physical, personal and social functioning. It is characterised by a state of deep sadness, loss of interest in activities usually felt as pleasant and an easy tiredness or lack of energy. Depression can affect people of all age groups, being more frequent in the elderly, it can be unexpected, recurrent or chronic, and lead to a substantial decrease in the individual's ability to carry out daily responsibilities (APA, 2000).

However, a small number of those affected receive adequate treatment, and the stigma weighs significantly on them. The way the population characterizes the symptoms of depression and the beliefs about its cause can interfere in the process of seeking help, the acceptance to treatment, as well as the attitude and behavior of society towards the carriers of this disorder. (BLAY; PELUSO; 2008; p.2).

When there is a strategy that allows physical activities and physical exercises to be performed in a planned and regular manner, the individual is prevented from going through mental suffering and, consequently, depression and has the opportunity to be included in social groups, enjoy self-esteem, improve cognitive functions and cope with the depressive mood. In addition, physical activity contributes to the prevention and treatment of common medical conditions in life and provide a better quality of life and social well-being to people.Having quality of life is not the absence of disease, but also reveal important factors such as longevity, job satisfaction, salary, leisure, family relationships, mood, pleasure and spirituality.(SANTANA; 2014; p. 21).

The aim of the research was to understand the importance of practicing physical exercises, accompanied and guided by professionals, adapting the activities for a better result, intensifying them according to the needs of each person and also to approach physical exercise as an alternative to combat depression.

- Enunciate concept and diagnosis of depression;
- Define difference between exercise and physical activity
- To recognise the promotion of quality of life for people with depressive disorder.
- Analyse forms of physical exercise for the treatment of depression;
- To know the effects of physical exercise in the socialisation process of depressed people.

WHAT IS DEPRESSION?

Depression is currently mentioned as the fourth mostpresent disease in the world. It is estimated that the disease has affected 121 million people, and less than 25% of the depressed obtain treatment. It is estimated that 5-10% of the world's population will have at least one episode of depression in their lifetime. Women are more likely to be depressed (10 to 20%) than men (5 to 12%). (BARBOSA; MARCEDO; SILVEIRA; 2011; p.7). According to Quintela (2010), people with depression have been experiencing a process of self-victimization and, at first, a possible disorder of their mental health.

The World Health Organization (WHO) has been studying the manifestations of depression for a long time. Depression has been analyzed by several health areas, and because it is conceived as a factor of great concern by scholars. And with technological advancement, and the rather fast pace of life, it makes people have less time to devote to their health. The results is a complex interchange between genetic and environmental events, which in turn, are related to a huge number of development of mental illnesses, there is an amount of approximately 450 million people affected by disorders worldwide, and that can be shown, from the threats faced in everyday life, the frustrations and stress that directly influence the diagnostic categorization of the listed pathologies (LEMOS and SOUZA, 2007 apudMaia, PEREIRA, MENEZES, 2015,p.180).

However mental health problems is one of the major causes of morbidity in today's societies with subsequent limitations. Most of them result in job loss due to unemployment and so on up to premature mortality. Some studies also developed in Portugal have recorded a strong correlation between depression, anxiety and stress. The comorbidity between depression and anxiety is very striking, and thus proving severity of symptoms.(APOSTOLO; et al; 2011; p.3)

Depression is considered one of the most frequent pathologies in the elderly, being classified as a chronic mental disorder that leads to a depressed mood, loss of interest and pleasure, feelings of guilt, sleep and appetite disturbances, decrease or loss of energy, difficulty concentrating, and thoughts of death and suicide.In the elderly, depression is mainly related to lifelong losses, declining health, deprivation, and social and economic aspects, therefore, it ends up being considered more common among people who are aging and is often not diagnosed or treated, and this age group receives the least incentive to treat it (SILVA et al, 2014a).

Symptoms of depression

The possibility of diagnosis may present several characteristics, from traits that comprise the daily experience of each individual, being the symptoms of depression reported by; (FERREIRA; 2017; p.14)

> [...] deep and prolonged sadness (in total more than two weeks), absence of motivation or enthusiasm in activities that were admired before, impression of emptiness, omission of energy, apathy, discouragement, absence of will to fulfil tasks, loss of expectation, negative, pessimistic reasoning, of accountability or self-devaluation. Besides these, the person may have blockages to concentrate, not sleep well, lack appetite, impatience and

> vague physical complaints (gastric discomfort, headache, among others). In more delicate occasions, thoughts of death and suicide may arise, and there are even people who attempt suicide. Depression is often a repetitive illness, the person has facts of depression that recur from moment to moment (NETO, 2010).

Because in face of the lay research around the mental disorders, and, on the other hand, the rapture of improper diagnoses that classified patients as having mental disorders, then there was the need to thoroughly construct the real symptoms that harm an individual with mental disorder. Health professionals (psychiatrists, psychologists) were able to better understand the action of the disorders through guidelines provided in diagnostic manuals. Thus, when treating the depressive disorder, the Diagnostic and Statistical Manual of Mental Disorders, (DSM-V, 5ª Edition, APA), points to the perspective that, in the face of so many changes in the lives of depressed people, they begin to reduce their social life with society and even with their families and closest people, and, it is from these reasons that suicidal thoughts may arise. (FERREIRA; 2017; p.15)

People who have experience with a person struck by depression can diagnose it just by observing the changes that the person begins to present. The depressed person starts to change their appearance from a happy person to a deeply sad person, begins to show lack of motivation to perform tasks that were part of their daily lives, with all this they begin to have thoughts of rejection, begin to devalue themselves thinking they are not able to do or be anything else, then finally the person starts to feel lack of appetite. (FERREIRA; 2017; p.15)

About 15% of the severely depressed commit suicide (WHO, 2002). According to the DSM-IV (Diagnostic and Statistical Manual of Mental Disorders, 4th edition), the fundamental characteristic of a major depressive event is a stage of at least two weeks during which there is a depressed mood or decreased interest or pleasure in almost all activities. In children and adolescents the mood may be irritable rather than sad. The individual must also experience at least four symptoms, which include:

changes in weight and appetite, sleep and psychomotor activity; loss of energy; feelings of abandonment or guilt; complications in thinking, concentrating or making decisions; recurrent thoughts about death or suicidal ideation, suicide plans or attempts. Depression is considered according to the criteria: mild, moderate and severe. In moderate and severe cases, it is always necessary to expose the presence of ideas about death or suicidal ideation (BARBOSA; MARCEDO; SILVEIRA; 2011; p.7).

In-service training programs are classified as stressful, and may stimulate the development of anxiety and depression, impairing health conditions, the quality of life of professionals and the quality of care provided to users of health services. (ROTTA ET AL., 2016; CARVALHO, MELO- FILHO, CARVALHO, & AMORIM, 2013; LOURENÇÃO ET AL., Elements such as the presence of severe patients and diseases, living with suffering and death, the pressure to make decisions, the fear of making mistakes, overwork and, often, the lack of appropriate infrastructure in health services cause fear among professionals, changing their performance and generating physical and emotional stress, such as anxiety and depression.

Depression is seen as one of the main reasons for disability worldwide. It can be long-term or recurrent, affecting people's efficiency at work and in daily life. It is considered that 350 million people are harmed by depression, and it is more frequent among women. It is determined by a confusion of sensations and changes in the individuals' behavior, such as sadness, loss of interest or pleasure, detachment from social activities, decrease of interest in professional, academic and play activities, loss of pleasure in interpersonal relationships, feeling of guilt or low self-esteem, sleep or appetite disturbances, tiredness lack of concentration (WORLD HEALTH ORGANIZATION [WHO], 2015).

Treatment of depression

The lifestyle of primitive civilisations included regular physical activity, in which there were irregular and continuous activities associated with hunting, farming and gathering in groups. Santos (2009). The probability of awakening biological factors in the recovery of the depressed individual are proven valid, being these of clear evidence, because they provide stimuli that become very important in the way the subject behaves in front of life; (FERREIRA; 2017; p.20)

> "Settling an objective view of some benefits of the application of physical exercises on a daily basis, we can mention several components: improvements in physiological aspects, such as reduction of harmful levels of bad cholesterol, help in controlling blood pressure, weight control, among others. Regarding the social aspects: possibility of experiential in movements with different cultural aspects, respect for rules, companionship during the ones that interact with different ones, besides dozens of other possibilities of addition to the practitioner" (COLOVINI, 2010, p.12).

Endorphins help relieve pain and also regulate our emotions. Running is a great example of physical exercise that has a high relationship of hormonal release, the endorphin is the main hormone released in the race, the same is a biochemical analgesic substance, ie, a natural painkiller, which has its construction in our body enhanced with physical exercises. For Ferreira (2012) even if there is inconstancy of temperament, the development of physical exercise can confirm expressive states of healthy temperament, the gradual addition of resistance of the individual in relation to psychosocial stressors. Considering that the same will have the opportunity to contain daily conflicts, from the involvement with physical exercises.

According to Benedetti et al (2008);

> [...] for the WHO the presence in light and moderate physical activities can delay functional decadence.

> Thus, an active life increases mental health and favours the management of disorders.

Hormones in the treatment of depression

According to Carvalho (2003) apud (2012);

> At the moment of adopting active ways of life, the person starts to gain daily the influence of well-being hormones such as endorphin and serotonin, can benefit their cardiorespiratory efficiency, muscle strength, flexibility, body awareness, also the enjoyment of the moment adopted for leisure, i.e. freedom in case of schedules and/or mandatory charges. (CARVALHO 2003, apudFERREIRA, 2012, P.9).

According to Hortencio (2008) "exercise may also be related to the composition of dopamine, due to an increase in calcium levels in the brain". The proposition found in bibliographies for the effectiveness of physical exercises as an incentive in the recovery from depression, potentially refers to the addition of flame substances, opioid catecholamines, being, serotonin,

For Moutri, Nunes and Bernik (2007) cited by Ferreira (2012),

> [...] when investigating exercise physiologically, it causes changes similar to those that the individual knows during a panic attack, that is, it could be the stressor gestor that will unleash a psychological-biological process of evaluation and reaction preparation (physiological changes), thus being able to favor for psychotherapeutic intervention with a successive and organized practice through specific physical training. What bases the search for the

understanding of the sets and psychophysiological effects of physical exercise on anxiety.

It is possible to identify in studies that the practice of acceptable physical activities has as a result the antidepressant effect, integrating as a preventive measure of anxiety, stress, and consequently the improvement of depression and insomnia. (IPAN, 2012). From this perspective, Ferreira (2012) highlights the importance of quality of life made possible by physical exercise, which includes emotional health, with direct action on self-esteem, enabling the individual to enjoy a healthy life, given that such factors promote the prolongation of life. To

In a study carried out Mathos, Andrade, Luft (2004) assess that,

> [...] among the variables in which the impact of physical activity was understood as "total effect", it can be conceptualized that there is a link between the improvement of the body figure and physical, psychological and social appearances. [...]. Being able to note the joint improvement of these variations through physical activity.

Depression prevention

In situations of prevention of depression, some possibilities are revealed, such as the treatment of people with mental problems; the adequate presentation of news and information about depression and suicides in the media and a necessary articulation of clinical and educational factors for populations at risk and in general. Health professionals in general have little knowledge about ways to detect cases of depression with suicide risk and the approach itself made in the care of people with suicide attempts.BARBOSA; MARCEDO; SILVEIRA; 2011; p.10)

Along their exposition, Stella et al. (2002) mention that physical activity is a preventive way of depressive symptoms. The authors argue that physical activity, when planned and practiced continuously, contributes to the reduction of the psychological suffering of the depressed individual. As it is likely to verify, the benefits of physical activity practice on psychological controls are practically sustained.

PHYSICAL EXERCISE AND PHYSICAL ACTIVITY

Physical activity depression

In order to avoid probable mistakes when conceptualizing the practice of physical exercise, the authors recommend classifying physical activity and physical exercise according to their specificities, which covers all body movement generated by skeletal muscles with energy expenditure above the levels of inactivity.MILES (2007) apud Santos (2009) points out that physical activity is a complex and multidimensional behavior. Among these, stands out as technical activities of occupational nature, and they are dedication to the house, recreational activities, with regard to the achievements made at times of leisure.

The Ministry of Health considers as "physical activity in leisure time" the performance of light or moderate intensity activity for 150 minutes per week; or vigorous intensity for at least 75 minutes per week (BRASIL, 2001).Shahbazzadeghan et al. (2010) show that the regular practice of physical activity generates benefits at both the physical and mental levels. At the latter level, the development of healthy social relationships and increased self-esteem can be evidenced.

Vidmar,et al (2011, p.418) point out that, in order to have a healthy lifestyle, it is necessary to include physical activity and certainly this can have an impact on people's quality of life. However, other healthy habits need to be developed, such as healthy eating, adequate sleep, weight control, among others. The same author also highlights a model of quality of life for the elderly, which encompasses "four conceptual dimensions: *behavioural competence, environmental conditions, perceived quality of life and subjective well-being".*

When explaining the physical exercise, the authors highlight it as being a programmed practice, which demands a previous structuring, because it has as intermediate or final objective, to promote to the individual a maintenance of his/her health and physical fitness. (CASPERSEN. POWELL. CHRISTENSON, 1985 apudCHEIK, 2003).In order to produce complementary forms to the functions offered to the physical exercise, TEIXEIRA, COSTA, MATSUDO, CORDAS (2008) point out in their work that, when accomplishing a planning of exercises, the performance must be based on the components that guarantee flexibility, posture and strength. Having in mind, the activities in teams, or properly the aerobic activities of moderate intensity. In this way, it is possible the construction or improvement of gains, which can be achieved in the guided practice of physical exercise.

Physical exercise is an option open to people's demand. It is affirmed that the practice is as an educational, playful, recreational, competitive, aesthetic character, and that it varies according to the place and objective for which it is firmed. Thus, it is adopted the general view that there is an exploration of physical abilities structured, achieving results based on different objectives. In view of this interpretation, the author points to the aprioristic reflections of each individual, in which there is a search for goals. The developments of healthy habits are proposals that must be achieved, therefore, such habits can integrate in the relations and motivations that the individual gets, actions must be adopted and modified throughout the practice, so that results can be achieved.(FERREIRA; 2017; p.17,18)

According to Rahal (2007, p. 86), "it is important to reveal that physical exercise is not just a series of exercises similar to those in the gym or the practice of sports activities". Physical exercise is considered a systematised sequence of movements of different body segments, executed in a planned way and with a certain objective to be achieved, such as the improvement or maintenance of physical fitness.

For Pescatelo (2004) the regular practice is known for its physical, psychological and social benefits, highlighting the improvement of strength, power and muscle flexibility; improvement of cardiorespiratory and cognitive performance; improved mobility; improved balance; prevention of bone mass loss; the reduction of functional disability, intensity of negative thoughts and physical illnesses and the promotion of well-being and mood are benefits of physical exercise and among others. Thus, we perceive that the practice of physical exercises minimizes physiological effects and the progression of chronic diseases, aspects that are typical of human aging.

All this favours the improvement of physical capacity; maintenance and recovery of independence, health and quality of life. Contributing to reducing the use of curative health services, medications, risk of development or worsening of chronic diseases, institutionalization and premature death (MACIEL, 2010). Such benefits are already demonstrated in several studies, cited in the following paragraphs, on the intervention of physical exercise when related to the non-drug control of depression, prevention of falls and improvement of quality of life in the elderly.In the elderly with depression, the benefits of physical exercise are also latent, since it influences the positive perception of self-image, self-esteem, reduces stress and anxiety, reduces depressive symptoms and increases social interaction, feelings of confidence and safety.(TEIXEIRA; 2017; SANTOS et al, 2014b; SILVA et al, 2014a; MELO et al, 2014; NOGUEIRA et al, 2014).

This study is justified due to the great worsening of depression that currently exists, thus altering the quality of life of many people around the world. The lack of awareness, information, motivation and even specific care makes depression one of the most disabling diseases in the world, limiting physical, personal and social functioning.

The depressed person needs adequate planning, including the regular practice of physical activity and exercise, a change in habits and a treatment that awakens the biological factors that help in the recovery of the depressed person.

There is still little knowledge of how to detect cases of depression. However, the use of antidepressants and psychotherapeutic monitoring, associated with physical activity when planned and regular, helps to reduce the psychological suffering of the depressed person, isolation and low self-esteem, thus occurring a gradual recovery.

METHODOLOGY

Study design: it will be characterized as being a literature review. This work was carried out in a descriptive way, where it seeks to describe the quality of life and physical exercise for the treatment of depression, where the explanation of the facts is exposed.

The research was conducted on well-known platforms such as Scielo, Google Scholar, Brazilian Journal of Physical Education, BVS and Berime, which form the database collected. Where the main objective was the population, which is being affected by this evil that is depression. The bibliographical survey was carried out in the period of March and April 2018. A total of 35 articles were selected.

All articles whose theme is pertinent to the study in question will be included. They will be free articles, published in the last 10 years, all in Portuguese. All articles that are not within the theme in question will be excluded. In total, 21 articles were excluded, being used 14 articles.

RESULTS AND DISCUSSION

Chart 1 - Description of the studies on the benefits of physical activity and exercise on the quality of life of people with depression

Author / Year / Journal	Type of study	Objective	Sample	Parameters used	Main results
Lucas Wederson De Souza Ferreira (2017) Faema	Literature review	Express the importance of physical exercise in the treatment of people with depression.	Not applicable	Analyse forms of physical exercise for the treatment of depression	It clearly defined depression, and showed that physical exercise is indeed of utmost importance for those who are affected by it, and that the planned practice of physical exercise can bring back to life a being that no longer sees the colour of joy in life.
João Luís Alves Apóstolo	Descriptivecorrelation	To analyse the point	A total of 343 users	To describe levels of	This study reveals that 40

(2011) Magazine		prevalence of depression, anxiety and	participated in the study. The average	depression, anxiety and stress in the	to 45% of the individuals surveyed
Latin American Nursing		stress in users of a CHC in a city in Northern Portugal, to analyze gender differences and the relationship between depression, anxiety, stress.	age was 43.82 years, SD=16.75, minimum 18 years, maximum 99 years.	users of an urban/rural health centre, to analyse gender differences and the comorbidity between depression, anxiety and stress.	present some degree of affective-emotional disorder. It should be underlined that around 20% present severe or very severe levels of anxiety and stress, and that around 12% present severe or very severe levels of depression.
Luana Liberato Martins (2017) Universidad e do Sul de Santa Catarina	Descriptive research	To identify the prevalence of anxiety and depression in male workers and the regular practice of physical exercise	The sample was composed of 53 male individuals, characterized as non-probabilistic intentional	Use of regular physical exercise in male workers, who have a prevalence of anxiety and depression.	For future studies, we suggest further research involving the prescription of physical exercise as a means of prevention and treatment for anxiety and depression, paying attention to which are the best exercises for this type of public, what is the best intensity to be used and what is the ideal frequency.
Fabiana de Oliveira Barbosa (2011) SBPH Journal	Scientific paper	The objective of this paper is to review the contributions in the last 10 years about the clinical characteristics of depression that are linked to the suicide outcome; the difficulties of detection by physicians of	Not applicable	To develop an action plan to encourage the practice of physical activity and healthy living habits among the elderly in the catchment area of the ESF Mozar Corrêa.	The greater the knowledge on the topic of depression and the risks of suicide, the greater the chances of prevention.

		depressive disorders; The lack of social support that makes adequate treatment difficult; the discussion and analysis of this phenomenon considered complex and multidimensional; and the prevention measures and adoption of strategies to address populations at risk for suicidal behaviour.			
Sérgio Luís Blay(2008) Revista Saúde Pública	Household survey	Assess how the population identifies symptoms of depression and its causes	The symptoms presented were identified as	Analysis of depression in the population of the city of São Paulo	The population of São Paulo in general and the people with the highest level of education
			"depression' by less than half of the sample. Around 20% of respondents believed it to be mental illness		in particular present a psychosocial model of depression that departs from the biomedical model.
Cláudia Gazetta (2017) Revista Portuguesa de Enfermage m de Mental Health,	Cross-sectional study	To evaluate the levels of anxiety and depression of professionals enrolled in the improvement and refinement programs of a public institution in the interior of the State of São Paulo.	The professionals present a profile of susceptibility to physical and emotional wearyness related to work - age bracket of 20 to 25 years (47.6), female (85.4%), single (90.2%). 46.8% of the professionals presented some degree of anxiety	Analysis of depression and anxiety in professionals who participate in improvement programmes.	The levels of anxiety and depression found are significant and show the presence of discouraging and/or stressful factors related to professional training in the evaluated programmes.

			and/or depression		
Francisca Elidivânia de Farias Camboim (2017) Revista de enfermage m UFPE online	Exploratory field study	describe the experience of the elderly with the benefits of physical activity for quality of life and cite the benefits of physical activity for the	Three categories emerged: a) Experiences of elderly women regarding the practice of physical activity; b) Benefits acquired with the	The use of physical activity to improve the quality of life of elderly people.	understands the importance of physical activity and all the aspects that permeate this practice in the process of ageing
		quality of life in old age	physical activity; c) Quality of life after adopting the practice of physical activity.		nto and in addressing this issue as health promotion and quality of life
Leilliane Fonseca Santana (2014) Federal University of Minas Gerais General	Literature review	To develop an action plan to encourage the practice of physical activity and healthy living habits in the elderly in the catchment area of the ESF Mozar Corrêa.	Not applicable	Elaboration of a project that works with the family and carers of the elderly, with the aim of providing information and knowledge about the ageing process.	Given the above, it is of utmost importance to implement policies that encourage an active life and, above all, that provide conditions for the inclusion of the elderly in society, reducing obstacles and increasing their access to health services.
F. Arbinaga(2 016) Cadernos de Psicologia do Esporte	Quantitative research	The present investigation aims to verify whether the practice of physical activity influences the self-esteem and the levels of depression in elderly people	The sample comprised 215 individuals (61 male and 154 female), practising and not practising physical activity, aged between 60 and 100 years.	The influence of physical activity on self-esteem and depression in elderly people.	In order to verify the normality of the data, the Skewness and Kurtosis values were analysed. It was found that for the self-esteem variable, the values are within the range of - 1 and 1, which was not verified for the depression variable
Erik Luiz Bonamigo (2017)	Descriptive study	To identify the presence of risk factors		To analyse the factors associated with	The importance of a follow-up for these people is

Catarinens and Medicine Archives		associated with depression in individuals with DM		depression in people with diabetes mellitus.	evident, in order to avoid both the evolution of the already established cases of diabetes-related depression and the development of new cases in patients who are in the early stages of the disease.
Renata Bernardi Rocha (2015) Federal University of Minas Gerais General	Literature review	To develop an intervention project to guide and encourage physical activity in the elderly in the coverage area of the blue team of the UBS Vila Cristina in the municipality of Betim / MG.	Not applicable	Use of physical activity for the prevention and promotion of health in the elderly.	The literature points out that regular physical activity is an important factor for the prevention and control of non-transmissible chronic diseases, besides keeping the elderly active, improving self-esteem, increasing social interaction, in short, providing a better quality of life.
Camila Oliveira de Moura Cabral (2017)	Qualitative study	Analyse motivational factors for participation of the elderly in a physical activity programme at the Convivência da Terceira Idade, in Teresina/PI.	The research subjects are 30 elderly people attended morning res of CCTI (Centro de Convivência da Terceira Idade / Rua Félix Pacheco, 152- Centro, Teresina- PI), aged 60 to 86 years old.	The contribution and motivation of physical exercise for the health and leisure of older people.	The practice of physical exercise is an important factor in the physical and psychosocial formation of the individual throughout his or her life, as the maintenance of a active and healthy lifestyle into old age is essential for the development of harmonious individual and social development.

Jessica de Nazaré Barbosa Teixeira (2017) UEPA	Quantitative approach	To evaluate the effects of physical exercise performed in a group of elderly in a UMS as a resource for prevention of health problems (depressive symptoms and risk of falls) and promotion of health, with emphasis on quality of life, as well as to evaluate their perception of these effects.	The study included the participation of 30 elderly individuals divided into two groups: G1, composed of 15 elderly who practiced physical exercise in the UMS and G2 composed of 15 elderly who did not practice physical exercise in Primary Health Care.	To identify the perception of the elderly regarding the effects of physical exercise performed in Primary Health Care as a resource for health promotion and protection.	We can conclude with this research that the practice of physical exercise performed in the Primary Health Care shows a strategy capable of not only stimulating, but also creating the opportunity for the elderly population to adopt a healthy lifestyle that leads to physical emancipation and the maintenance of functional capacity,
					resulting in a better quality of life for this population.
Làzaro Rivera Valido (2016) Universidad e Federal De Minas General	Intervention study	Elaborate an intervention proposal to promote improvement in the quality of life of the elderly in the catchment area of the Family Health Strategy Family (ESF) of the Amaro Lanari, Coronel Fabriciano, Minas Gerais, through the systematic practice of supervised physical activities	Not applicable	Raise awareness of the ESF team professionals about the importance of disseminating information on the positive effects on physical and mental health through the systematic practice of physical activities	he need to make the elderly aware of the importance of their participation in physical activities, in order to improve their quality of life, their degree of independence and autonomy and, consequently, their citizenship.

PHYSICAL EXERCISE AND PHYSICAL ACTIVITY

Physical activity is any body movement that is made through musculoskeletal contraction, and that has an energy expenditure in the body. On the other hand, physical exercise is an activity properly planned and structured according to the individual's need and ability, in order to improve or maintain one or more components of physical fitness (ACSM, 2009).One of the ways to manage stress (and consequently depression and anxiety) is the practice of physical activities from mild to moderate, which comprises regular physical exercise and fitness improvement (NAHAS, 2013).

According to the Ministry of Health (2016), the practice of physical activities is good for the mind and body. The practice of regular physical activity is indicated for people of all ages, both as a preventive activity, in healthy people, and therapeutically, in debilitated people. The benefits of the practice for the individual's health, besides enabling the maintenance and/or elimination of body mass, reduces the risk of heart disease, hypertension, stroke, cancer, diabetes, strengthens bones and muscles, reduces stress, anxiety and depression, improves mood and stimulates social interaction.(MARTINS; 2017; p.3).

Regular exercises, besides bringing physiological benefits, cause psychological benefits, such as a better impression of well-being, mood and self-esteem. For the clinical plan, physical activity produces beneficial emotional effects in any age and gender (COSTA; SOARES; TEIXEIRA, 2007). According to Knapenet al. (2015), health professionals should be informed of the various characteristics of depression. Especially among physical education and physiotherapy professionals, motivational strategies should also be added in the form of physical exercises to increase adherence and motivation of individuals/patients in specific training or rehabilitation programs, which makes this analysis valuable for the areas.

The accession of mental health associated with physical activity is an area that has been seen as one of the possibilities of action of this professional. The little scientific knowledge about the mental health associated, many times, to the little time of practical experience of the professionals of physical education generates the absence of a bigger knowledge about the psychological benefits of the physical activity on these pathologies. (MATTOS; ANDRADE; LUFT, 2004)

The physical education professional has many challenges and responsibilities, needing to be always informed/updated about various contents so that he/she can incorporate them to his/her work in a profitable way, having the opportunity to act in a competent way. In the same line of understanding, it is worth noting that the academics and physical education professionals should be ready to deal with people who have different characteristics and the knowledge of some diseases and thus improve their possibilities of acting, improving the chances of success when dealing with people assaulted by depression and anxiety. (MARTINS; 2017; p.3)

According to Camelo (2008), mediations to promote beneficial results to the worker at psychological and physiological levels are very important to reduce the effects of stressful events at work. The author states that, in the literature, there are studies that point to the fact that the tensions caused by work, the stress levels and the diseases caused by this, can be minimised through the practice of physical activity.

For Hassmen, Koivula and Uutela (2000), place that complex levels of sense of coherence and social integration are notable in individuals who exercise at least twice a week the frequent physical exercise brings physiological and psychological benefits, and therefore is a positive health behavior. Regarding the effect of exercise for mental health, there are increasing features that it brings benefits for the interversion of mental illness, however it can be stated that it is still not customary for psychologists to habitually use physical exercise as part of treatments.(AMERICAN PSYCHOLOGICAL ASSOCIATION, 2017).

According to the Federal Council of Physical Education (CONFEF, 2004), one of the main options in the search for good health is the practice of physical activity. Besides relieving stress, it makes the body release beta-endorphin, promoting a sense of well-being, sleep improvement and causes a feeling of relaxation. Sanches et al. (2016)complement by stating that physical exercise is a non-pharmacological means used to prevent, avoid and/or control chronic stress and its benefits incorporate an improvement in emotional state and in the individual's lipid and glycemic control.

According to CONFEF (2004) and Hassmén, Koivula and Uutela (2000), people who exercise two to three times a week are less affected by depression, stress, anger and distrust when compared to those who do not exercise or exercise less frequently. People have already discovered that physical exercise makes their day more pleasant and they seek changes in their life habits through the practice of it. These changes are reflected on the emotional side, reversing depression and improving self-esteem.

Brunoniet al. (2015), state that the prescription of strength training based on the perception of effort is an effective method for a reduction in depressive symptoms in the elderly and also improves the quality of life related to health. In an investigation with depressed elderly women, they concluded that after strength training, there was a reduction in depressive symptoms and their frequency. In addition, improvements were seen in functional capacity, general health status, mental health and vitality.

According to Salmon (2001), researches point out that aerobic training exerts anxiolytic and antidepressive effects and protects individuals from the harmful effects of stress on physical and mental health. For the author, there is evidence that exercise imposes lasting resistance to stress. For the *Association for Applied Sport Psychology* (2017) a short walk and/or 10 minutes of aerobic exercise are already sufficient for mood improvement and increased energy and long-term benefits. Exercise promotes psychological benefits and generates better ability to cope with stress. According to the association, the ideal is to exercise 30 minutes, three times a week at a moderate intensity. Programs longer than 10 weeks work best for reducing depressive symptoms.

Woolston (2016) notes that in fact, in order to improve mood through physical exercises, it is simply to try to find a modality that the person really likes that gives him pleasure, such as joining a walking group, in which one will have social benefits, besides the exclusion of the need to get any special equipment. According to CONFEF (2017), researches prove that physical activity helps to improve diseases and especially mood, and thus, It fights stress, anxiety and depression, changing the individual's life and even reducing or abandoning the routine of medications in several situations. They also reduce sedentary lifestyles, as well as pain, anxiety and stress symptoms, and improve sleep and immunity.

Gonçalves (2016) found, in a study in a health centre with adults about the difficulties to practice physical exercise, that the most frequent reasons were the "long working day" (44.55%), the "family commitments" (40.59%) and the "housework" (31.68%), i.e., the lack of time also emerges as one of the biggest impediments to the practice of physical exercise. It seems that lack of time is a problem that modernity will need to learn to manage so as not to have losses and complications in their health. Therefore, this study indicates that a better formation of daily priorities associated with a good organization of time may increase the rates of physical exercise and decrease physical inactivity.

According to Telles et al. (2016), many people prefer not to exercise, alleging, among other reasons, lack of time, lack of motivation, the need to approach a gym (lack of transportation, crowded gyms, and lack of closer gyms), loss of energy, health problems, and lack of money. According to Moraes et al. (2007), depression decreases the practice of physical activities and at the same time, physical activity is essential in the prevention and treatment of depression, especially in those who have advanced age.

The indispensable problems of the application of physical exercise as a treatment are: the initial acceptance and the adherence of discouraged individuals to exercise regimes, issues that require dedication.(SCHUCH; FLECK, 2013).Epidemiological studies prove that exercise and physical activity, besides showing therapeutic benefits, prevent or delay several mental disorders, such as anxiety, eating and affective disorders.In addition, habitual physical activity increases the release of hormones and neurotransmitters being these producers of the sense of well-being (CONFEF, 2017).

In 2020, the World Health Organization (WHO) predicts that depression will be the second reason for absence from work due to illness in the world, and unemployment is a major threat factor for work-related depression (JARDIM, 2011). This data reinforces the importance of encouraging the practice, because according to Andrade (2011, p.3), "in recent decades, studies have shown that physical exercises can also collaborate in the improvement of depressive conditions".

In reducing depressive signs and cognitive performance, the benefits of physical activity can be understood in three levels of intervention: primary intervention, which protects health and prevents the onset of diseases, which decreases the risk of depression, cognitive decline and dementia; secondary intervention, which identifies the disease in advance and seeks to treat it, since mild cognitive impairment and depression can be overcome with physical activities; tertiary intervention, which prevents the progression of the disease, treating its symptoms.(COELHO; VIRTUOSO, 2014).

Given this, the practice of physical activities offers adult and elderly individuals several benefits that go beyond health promotion, by promoting well-being.and improve social relationships of the elderly giving them leisure activities. (CABRAL et al; 2017; p.10). Schuch and Fleck (2013) state that meta-analyses demonstrate that physical exercise has similar objective to other treatments used for depression, such as the intake of some antidepressants and psychotherapies. Therefore, for the authors, exercise is neither less nor more effective than traditional treatments. (MARTINS; 2017; p.16)

Gain in quality of life

Nahas (2006) apud Silva (2012) sees the various possibilities that may associate and contribute to life expectancy, in terms of quantity and quality of years lived, including some factors, such as the genetic influence, environmental variations and the various causes in human behaviour. In the midst of all conceptions which encompass quality of life, it is essential to search for means which help the subject to achieve well-being. However, an obstacle is found, when the subject is assaulted by the depressive disorder, and how the same reacts to the charges of everyday life. (FERREIRA; 2017; p.19)

According to Matos (1996) apud Silva (2012) in a dialogue that has as stimulus to talk about Quality of Life, it is inconceivable that it is not of interest the human motivation, because it is so that the human being has the possibility to seek and discover with their needs, so that they can design a path to achievement. According to Ferreira (2017) in the midst of all the concepts that cover the quality of life, it is essential to search for means that help the subject to achieve their well-being.

The word Quality of Life includes the physical, social, psychological and spiritual development of individuals. The physical is defined by functional activity, strength, tiredness, sleep, rest, pain and other symptoms. Social well-being is related to affectivity, entertainment, work, economic situation and family suffering. The psychological shows up through fear, anxiety, depression and anguish, which can lead to illness and, finally, the spiritual, which has its concept based on aspects such as hope, uncertainty, religiosity and inner strength. (CAMBOIM et al; 2017; p.2)

Some authors point out quality of life as being the level of satisfaction with life, in which it needs the connection of several factors, such as habits of life, physical activity, perception of well-being, physical and environmental conditions, family relationships and friendship (NERI, 2001).Quality of life, according to the definition of the World Health Organisation (WHO), is related to the complexity of the interaction between physical health, psychological state, level of dependence, social relationships, beliefs and relationship with the environment.

Rodrigues and Lara (2011) further add to this definition the personal well-being, functional capacity, socioeconomic level, self-care and family support of the individual. They also specify that, in aging, quality of life represents the maintenance of health in all aspects of human life (physical, social, psychological and spiritual), well-being, personal satisfaction and prosperity in aging. Quality of life is socially represented through objective and subjective values. Especially if we take into consideration issues related to happiness, love, well-being, pleasure or personal fulfillment or else, if we consider material, cultural, social assets, among others that contribute to the analysis of concepts about quality of life. (VALIDO; 2016; p. 19)

Depression as a factor aggravating quality of life

For Noble, Greene, Levinson et al (2001) apud Berber, Kupek, Berber (2004) in the situation of the depressed, there is a worsening in social and emotional function, because depressed patients return to isolate themselves from some relationship, and show behaviors such as some frustrations as: disappointment, grief and losses. However, the various means of recognising the depressed subject, either through their behaviour, or through diagnoses or infamy, have been prepared and are currently in conformity with the factors that relate to the way in which sufferers of depression relate to other human beings. In this way they feel unable to develop any kind of relationship with other people.

For Berber, Kupek, Berber (2004), "Depression considerably worsens physical fitness, physical functioning, social functioning and emotional functioning, and potentially affects mental health". Given what was indicated above, it is visible in the reports of the authors that depression eventually harms the life of the individual, if untreated, so that the depressed subject tends to seek social isolation, having low self-esteem as the main aspect. (FERREIRA; 2017; p.19)

In the search for treatment for depressive disorder, there are several ways researched by the sciences, from the use of antidepressants associated with psychotherapy. When the treatment is carried out through the use of medication, there is a gradual recovery, and in a few weeks results are already obtained, which protects against new depressive crises. However, in the psychotherapeutic monitoring cutting the use of medication, the patient's recovery is much more effective, so in the function of the two treatment procedures, there is a complement of gains in recovery, in which the depressed person alters considerably the relationship with other people, and thus expressing affection. (NETO; 2010).

Quality of life at work

Most companies have been seeking to ally their structure and organization within internal work, and in ways that encourage the presence of healthy lifestyle habits, such as good nutrition, frequency of physical activity practice, time and quality of adequate sleep/rest, among others (FIGUEIREDO; MONT'ALVÃO, 2008).Pereira (2014) states as to stress symptoms, the main symptoms identified in order of importance in a global sample were anxiety, nervousness, fatigue, irritability for no apparent reason, distress and pain in the neck and shoulder muscles. That the causes of tension at work that most explain stress are the day full of work commitments undertaken, little or no free time, end up not being able to disconnect from the work-related situation.

Quality of life and physical activity

Physical activity plays an important role in Quality of Life being ahead in the actions and programs composed in the Family Health Strategies (FHS) as health promotion and prevention of chronic diseases allowing people longevity and well-being. The practice of physical activity is an essential benefit to bodily and mental health, especially in old age, when the functional capacity suffers reduction and the body weakens becoming sensitive to the increase of diseases. (CAMBOIM et al; 2017; p.2). Therefore, the benefits of physical activity together, make it provides active people more health, and consequently a better quality of life.

Quality of life and physical exercise

Miranda (2003) announces strong evidence that physical exercise is still the best way to maintain and preserve life and health at any age, benefiting your quality of life, i.e. feeling good in the best possible way. Thus, Kolowsky (2004) determines quality of life as being a person's degree of satisfaction with life. In this situation, the activities that provide well-being, satisfaction and leisure are fundamental in the construction of a life with quality.

When relating physical exercise and quality of life, it is possible to see the close relationship between the benefits of exercise and the improvement of physical, psychological and social domains in both the quality of life questionnaires and the self-reports of the elderly (EIRAS et al., 2010). Studies show that older people who engage in regular physical exercise have better quality of life indices when compared to older people who do not exercise. This is because, by improving and maintaining autonomy, functionality, physical fitness, the adoption of a healthy lifestyle, contribute decisively in the quality of life of the elderly (TORRES et al, 2010; CAMPOLINA; DINI; CICONELLI, 2011; RODRIGUES; LARA, 2011; SILVA et al, 2012a).

CONCLUSION

We conclude with this work that the person with depression has at first a mental disorder, and may have a process of self-victimization, generated by frustrations and stress caused by the fast pace of life. The depressed person seeks activities that provide satisfaction, building the foundations for a life with more quality.

Through physical activity, which is an occupational activity that can be recreational or performed during leisure time, one can prevent and treat depressive symptoms and thus contribute to reduce the psychological suffering of the depressed person. On the other hand, physical exercise is a programmed practice, which aims to promote the maintenance of health and physical fitness, making the person to consider again issues related to happiness, love, well-being, pleasure and personal fulfilment, leaving behind social isolation and low self-esteem. It is possible to diagnose a person with depression, just by observing some changes that the person starts to present and thus help him/her to look for a specific treatment.

BIBLIOGRAPHIC REFERENCES

ACSM - American College of Sports Medicine (Position Stad) Exercise and physical activity for older adults. **Medicine and Science in Sports and Exercise**, V. 47, n. 7, p. 1510 - 1530, 2009.

AMERICAN PSYCHOLOGICAL ASSOCIATION.**The exercise effect**.2011. Available at: <http://www.apa.org/monitor/2011/12/exercise.aspx>.

ANDRADE, T. **Physical exercise in the treatment of depression: a literature review**. 2011. 30f. Course Conclusion Paper (Graduation in Physical Education). School of Physical Education. State University of Campinas, Campinas, 2011.

APA (2002). DSM-IV-TR - Diagnostic and Statistical Manual of Disorders

mentais - 4° edição. Lisbon: Climepsi.

APÓSTOLO, JOÃO LUÍS ALVES; FIGUEIREDO, MARIA HENRIQUETA; MENDES, AIDA CRUZ;

RODRIGUES, MANUEL ALVES; Depression, anxiety and stress in primary health care users.**Revista Latino-Americana.**Enfermagem [INTERNET]. Mar-abr 2011.

ASSOCIATION FOR APPLIED SPORT PSYCHOLOGY.**Psychological Benefits of Exercise.**Available at: <http://www.appliedsportpsych.org/resources/health-fitness- resources/psychological-benefits-of-exercise/>.

BARBOSA, FABIANA DE OLIVEIRA; MARCEDO, PAULA COSTA MOSCA; SILVEIRA, ROSA MARIA CARVALHO; **Depression and Suicide**; Rev. SBPH vol.14 no.1, Rio de Janeiro - Jan/Jun. - 2011.

BENEDETTI, T, R, B. et al. **Physical activity and mental health status of the elderly**. Rev Saúde Pública 2008.

BERBER, JOANA DE SOUZA, SANTOS KUPERK, EMIL BERBER, SAULO CAÍRES. Prevalence of Depression and its Relationship with Quality of Life in Patients with Fibromyalgia Syndrome. RevBrasReumatol, v. 45, n. 2, p. 47-54, mar./apr., 2005.

BLAY, SÉRGIO LUÍS; PELUSO, ÉRICA DE TOLEDO PIZA; Perception of depression by the population of the city of São Paulo; Botucatu-São Paulo; 2008.

BRASIL, Ministério da Saúde (MS). Avaliação de efetividade de programas de atividade física no Brasil. **Secretaria de Vigilância em Saúde**. Brasília, 2001.

BRUNONI, L. et al. Strength training decreases depressive symptoms and improves health-related quality of life in elderly women. **Revista Brasileira de Educação Física e Esporte**. São Paulo, v.29, n.2, p.189-196, jun. 2015. Available at: <http://www.scielo.br/scielo.php?script=sci_arttext&pid=S1807-55092015000200189&lng=en&tlng=en>.

CABRAL, CAMILA OLIVEIRA DE MOURA; COSTA, FÁBIO SOARES; SANTOS, ANDREIA MENDES; Elderly and physical exercise: motivations and contributions to health and leisure; Licere, Belo Horizonte, v.20, n.4, Dec/2017; 2017.

CAMBOIM, FRANCISCA ELIDIVÂNIA DE FARIAS; CAMBOIM, JOSÉ CLESTON ALVES; DAVIM, REJANE MARIE BARBOSA; NÕBREGA, MARIE OLIVEIRA; NUNES, ROSA MARTHA VENTURA; OLIVEIRA, SILVIA XIMENES; Benefits of physical activity in the elderly for quality of life; **Nursing Journal;** Recife; 2017.

CAMELO, S. Psychosocial risks at work that can lead to stress: a literature review. **CiencCuidSaude.** V.7, n.2, p.232-240, abr/jun. 2008. Available at: <http://eduem.uem.br/ojs/index.php/CiencCuidSaude/article/viewFile/5010/3246>.

CARVALHO, C. N., MELO-FILHO, D. A., CARVALHO, J. A. G., & AMORIM, A. C. G. (2013). Prevalência e fatores associados aos transtornos mentais comuns em residentes médicos e da área multiprofissional. Jornal Brasileiro de Psiquiatria, 62(1), 38-45. doi: 10.1590/S0047- 20852013000100006

CASPERSEN, C., POWELL, K. & CHRISTENSON, G. (1985). Physical activity, exercise and physical fitness: Definitions and distinctions for healthrelated research.*Public Health Reports, 100,* 126-131.

COELHO, F.; VIRTUOSO, J. Atividade Física e Saúde Mental do Idoso. **Revista Brasileira de Atividade Física e Saúde**. Pelotas, v.19, n.6, p.663-664, nov. 2014.

COLOVINI, L. **Physical education and the promotion of mental health: systematic review of articles between 2000 and 2010.** 2010. 30f. Course Conclusion Paper (Physical Education Course: Graduation) - Federal University of Rio Grande do Sul. Porto Alegre, 2010.

CONFEF. **Physical activity is the path to a healthy life, guides physical educator.** Available at: < http://www.confef.org.br/extra/clipping/view.asp?id=1077>.

COSTA, R.; SOARES, H.; TEIXEIRA, J. Benefits of physical activity and physical exercise in depression. **Revista do Departamento de Psicologia**. Niterói, v.19, n.1, p.269-276, jun 2007. Available at: <http://www.scielo.br/pdf/rdpsi/v19n1/22.pdf>.

Cheik, C. N.E. et .Al. **Effects of physical exercise and physical activity on depression and anxiety in elderly individuals**. R. bras. Ci. e Mov. 2003; 11(3): 45-52.

EIRAS, S. B. et al. Factors of adherence and maintenance of physical activity practice by the elderly. Rev. Bras. Cienc. Esporte, Campinas, v. 31, n. 2, p. 75-89, January 2010. Available at: http://www.rbceonline.org.br/revista/index.php/RBCE/article/view/705/410

FERREIRA, LUCAS WEDERSON DE SOUZA; The importance of physical exercise in the treatment of people with depression, the evil of the century; Ariquemes-Rondônia; 2017.

FERREIRA, A, M. **Influence of physical exercise practice in stress. Article presented to the specialization course in bodybuilding and personal training of the centre for advanced studies and**

integrated training, endorsed by the pontifical catholic university of Goiás, 2012.

FIGUEIREDO, F.; MONT'ALVÃO, C. Ginástica Laboral e Ergonomia. 2. ed. Rio de Janeiro: Sprint, 2008.

GONÇALVES, C. **Barriers to physical exercise in leisure time among adult users of a Health Centre.** 2016. 46f. Mestrado integrado em medicina. Faculty of Medicine, University of Coimbra. Portugal, 2016.

HASSMÉN, P.; KOIVULA, N.; UUTELA, A. PhysicalExerciseandPsychologicalWell-Being: A PopulationStudy in Finland. **Preventive Medicine**. V.30, n.1, p.17-25, Jan 2000. Available at: <http://www.sciencedirect.com/science/article/pii/S0091743599905972>.

HORTENCIO ,R, F, H. et al. **Physical exercises in combating depression: perception of psychology professionals.** Published in 2008.

INSTITUTE FOR ADVANCED RESEARCH IN NEUROSTIMULATION (IPAN). **The importance of physical activity in the prevention of depression**. 10 de Agos. 2012.

JARDIM, S. Depression and work: rupture of the social bond. **Revista Brasileira de Saúde Ocupacional**. São Paulo, v.36, n.123, p.84-92, 2011. Available at: <https://www.fasul.edu.br/portal/app/webroot/files/links/Seguran%C3%A7a%20Trabalho/RBSO/RBSO%20123%20vol%2036.pdf#page=86>.

KNAPEN, J. et al. Exercise therapy improves both mental and physical health in patients with major depression. **Journal Disability and Rehabilitation.**V.37, n.16, p.1490- 1495.2015.Availablelem: <http://www.tandfonline.com/doi/citedby/10.3109/09638288.2014.972579?scroll=top&needA ccess=true>.

KOLOWSKY, M. Influências da atividade física no aumento da qualidade de vida. EFDeportes, v. 10, n. 69, 2004.

LOURENÇÃO, L. G., MOSCARDINI, A. C., & SOLER, Z. A. S. G. (2013). Quality of life of non-medical resident professionals.Journal of Nursing UFPE on line, 7(11), 6336- 6345.doi: 10.5205/reuol.3794-32322-1-ED.0711201304

MACIEL, M. G. Atividade física e funcionalidade do idoso. **Motriz**, Rio Claro, v.16, n.4, p.1024-1032, out.-dez. 2010. Accessed on: 07/09/2014, 11:57h. Available at: http://www.scielo.br/pdf/motriz/v16n4/a23v16n4.pdf.

MAIA, J, A. PEREIRA, L, A. MENEZES, F, A. Análise de fatores depressivos no trabalho do enfermeiro na área de psiquiatria. Revista SUSTINERE, Rio de Janeiro, v. 3, n. 2, p. 178190, jul-dez, 2015.

MARTINS, LUANA LIBERATO; Prevalence of anxiety and depression in male workers and the regular practice of physical exercise; Palhoça- Santa Catarina; 2017.

MATHOS, A, S. ANDRADE, A. LUFT, C, Di B. The contribution of physical activity in the treatment of depression. **Revista Digital** - Buenos Aires - Year 10 - N° 79 -December 2004. Available at:<http://www.efdeportes.com/efd79/depres.htm>.

MORAES, H. et al. Physical exercise in the treatment of depression in the elderly: a systematic review. **Revista de Psiquiatria do Rio Grande do Sul**. Porto Alegre, v.29, n.1, p.70-79, abr 2007. Available at: <http://www.scielo.br/pdf/rprs/v29n1/v29n1a14>.

MIRANDA, M. L. J. Música, atividade física e bem-estar psicológico em idosos. Revista Brasileira Ciência e Movimento, v. 4, n. 11, p. 87-94, 2003.

NAHAS, M. Atividade **física, Saúde e Qualidade de vida:** Conceitos e Sugestões para um Estilo de Vida Ativo, ed.6. Londrina: Midiograf, 2013.

NERI. A. L. Desenvolvimento e Envelhecimento: Perspectivas biológicas, psicológicas e sociológicas. São Paulo: Papirus, 2001.

NETO, M, R. L. Diseases: Depression (Depressive Disorder). Available at: < http://www.saudemental.net/depressao.htm>. Last Update: September/2010.

NOGUEIRA, E. L. et al. Screening for depressive symptoms in the elderly in the Family Health Strategy, Porto Alegre. Rev Saúde Pública, v. 48, n. 3, p. 368- 377. 2014. Accessed on: 28/09/2014, 17:28h. Available at: http://www.revistas.usp.br/rsp/article/view/84386

PESCATELO, L. S. Exercise and hypertension.American College of Sports Medicine Position Stand.Medicine Science Sports Exercices, v. 3, n. 36, 2004.

PEREIRA, L. Stress at work: a challenge for managers in Brazilian organizations. **REGE - Revista de Gestão.**

São Paulo, v.21, n.3, p.401-413, sep. 2014. Available at: <http://www.sciencedirect.com/science/article/pii/S1809227616301916>.

RAHAL, Miguel Antônio *et al.* **Physical activity for the elderly and objectives.** In:

PAPALÉO NETTO, Matheus; Tratado de Gerontologia. 2. ed. Rev. e ampl. São Paulo: Atheneu, 2007. P. 86-87.

RODRIGUES, AC..C; LARA, M.O. Qualidade de vida do idoso: um levantamento da produção científica nos últimos dez anos. R. Enferm. Cent. O. Min,v.1 ,n.3 , p. 395- 406, jul- sep. 2011. Accessed on: 07/09/2014, 17:44h. Available at: http://www.seer.ufsj.edu.br/index.php/recom/article/viewArticle/70

ROTTA, D. S., PINTO, M. H., LOURENÇÃO, L. G., TEIXEIRA, P. R., GONSALEZ, E. G., & GAZETTA, C. E. (2016). Levels of anxiety and depression among multiprofessional health residents. Revista Rene, 17(3), 372-377.

SANCHES, A. et al. Relationship among stress, depression, cardiovascular and metabolic changes and physical exercise. **Fisioterapia em Movimento**. Curitiba, v. 29, n.1, p.23-36, mar 2016. Available at: <http://www.scielo.br/scielo.php?script=sci_arttext&pid=S0103- 51502016000100023&lang=en>.

SALMON, P. Effects of Physical Exercise on Anxiety, Depression and Sensitivity to Stress - A Unifying Theory.**ClinicalPsychologyReview**. v.21, n.1, p.31-61, feb. 2001.

SANTANA, Leilliane Fonseca; Physical activity and its importance in the health and quality of life of the elderly; Uberaba- Minas Gerais; 2014.

SANTOS, A, L, P, S. **The relationship between physical activity and quality of life**. Thesis submitted to the School of Physical Education and Sports of the University of São Paulo as partial requirement for obtaining the degree of Doctor of Physical Education. SÃO PAULO 2009.

SANTOS, C. T. B. Envelhecimento no Brasil: da formulação de políticas à estruturação de serviços de saúde integrais. **Tempus Actas de Saúde Coletiva**, 2014.Disponívelem:http://www.tempusactas.unb.br/index.php/tempus/article/view/1454

SCHUCH, F.; FLECK, M. Is Exercise an Efficacious Treatment for Depression? A Comment upon Recent Negative Findings.**Frontiers in Psychiatry**.v.4, n.20, p.1-3, apr. 2013.Available at:

<https://www.ncbi.nlm.nih.gov/pmc/articles/PMC3613866/>.

SHAHBAZZADEGHAN, B., FARMANBAR, R., GHANBARI, A. & ROSHAN, Z. (2010).The study of the effects of the regular exercise program on the self-esteem of the elderly in the old people home of rasht. *EuropeanJournalof Social Sciences, 13*(2), 271- 277.

SILVA, WENDER, AFONSO. Physical activity and third age: a case study on the activities offered by the group Living Happy, the city of Beautiful Waters of Goias. Monograph Paper presented as a final requirement for approval in the discipline Course Completion Work II of the Degree in Physical Education Program Pro-Legree, Ceilândia - DF, 2012

SILVA, F.R. et al. Indicadores antropométricos e o risco de desenvolvimento de doenças cardiovasculares em um grupo de idosos praticantes de exercício físico. In: VII CONNEPI (North-Northeast Congress of Research and Innovation). Palmas, Tocantins, 2012a.

STELLA, F., GOBBI, S., CORAZZA, D.& COSTA, J. (2002). Depression in the elderly: Diagnosis, treatment and benefits of physical activity. Motriz, 8(3), 91-98

TEIXEIRA, Jessica de Nazaré Barbosa; Physical exercise applied to the elderly as a resource for health promotion in primary health care; Belém- Pará; 2016.

TEIXEIRA, C, P; COSTA, F, R; MATSUDO, M, M, S; CORDAS, A, T. The practice of physical exercise in patients with eating disorders. Revista de Psiquiatria Clínica, v.36, n.4, p.145-152, 2009. Digital Library of Intellectual Production - BDPI, University of São Paulo.

TELLES, T. et al. Adesão e aderência ao exercício: Um Estudo Bibliográfico. **Revista Brasileira de Psicologia do Esporte.** V.6, n.1. 2016. Available at: <https://portalrevistas.ucb.br/index.php/RBPE/article/view/6725/4286>. Accessed on: 01 Oct. 2017.

VALIDO, Lázaro Rivera; Benefits of the systematic practice of physical exercises in a group of elderly in the community of amaro lanari in the municipality coronel Fabriciano; Ipatinga- Minas Gerais ;2016.

VIDMAR, M. F. *et al.* Physical activity and quality of life in the elderly. **Ver. Saúde e Pesquisa**,v.4,n.3,2011.Available at:<http://periodicos.unicesumar.edu.br/index.php/saudpe

sq/article/viewFile/1714/1394>.

WOOLSTON, C. **DepressionandExercise.** Available at: <http://consumer.healthday.com/encyclopedia/depression-12/depression-news- 176/depression-and-exercise-648415.html>. Accessed on: 01 Oct. 2017.

WORLD HEALTH ORGANIZATION.(2015). Mental disorders.Accessed at http://www.who.int/mediacentre/factsheets/ fs396/en/

ZSCHUCKE, E.; GAUDLITZ, K.; STROHLE, A. Exercise and Physical Activity in Mental Disorders: Clinical and Experimental Evidence. **Journal of Preventive Medicine & Public Health**.v.46, suppl.1, p.12-21, Jan 2013. Available at:
<https://www.ncbi.nlm.nih.gov/pmc/articles/PMC3567313/#B22>.

CHAPTER 3

PERFORMANCE OF PHYSIOTHERAPY IN PATIENTS UNDERGOING MASTECTOMY

ISABEL CRISTINA BARBOSA DANTAS [1]
ROSA MARIA DA SILVA[1]
ANDRÉA LIMA DE SÁ[2]

Breast cancer is one of the most common neoplasms and with a high mortality rate, as it is the type that causes most death in the female population and the first in number of surgeries performed in Brazil per year (GIACON et al., 2013).

It is defined as a complex, heterogeneous disease, of unknown etiology, with high incidence and mortality, resulting in the formation of a malignant tumor from the excessive and disordered multiplication of abnormal cells, which presents itself through different clinical and morphological forms, with a high degree of tumor aggressiveness and high potential for metastasis. Therefore, there are types of breast cancer, which are the most common ductal carcinoma, lobular carcinoma, which affects both breasts and is less common, and the rarer inflammatory carcinoma, which is aggressive and affects the whole breast (LEONEL; BARBOSA; MACHADO, 2017).

In terms of incidence, breast cancer is the most frequent type among women in Brazil, with estimates of 28.1% per 100,000 women of all cases in 2016, totalling 57,960 cases. In the Northeast Region the estimate is 20.5% per 100,000 women, with a total of 11,190 cases (INCA, 2016).

The treatment for breast cancer consists of multiple interventions, mastectomy, chemotherapy, radiotherapy and hormone therapy. In the case of mastectomy, this is a surgery that depends on the degree of evolution of the tumour. When the disease is diagnosed, it shows its different stages, from the simplest to the most advanced state, which requires treatment through partial mastectomy or radical mastectomy (LEONEL; BARBOSA; MACHADO, 2017; GIACON et al., 2013).

Radical mastectomy is a non-conservative surgery, when extirpation of the breast, pectoral muscle, thoracic fascia and ipsolateral axillary lymph nodes occurs. It also involves part of the nerve supply to the thorax and shoulder muscles which may be disturbed. As for partial mastectomy, it is the breast-conserving surgery, which consists of the removal of only one quadrant of the breast (SOUZA; SOUZA, 2014).

In its complexity, mastectomy causes great fear among women, because, even being efficient, it is a surgical procedure that culminates in postoperative complications, with psychological changes, scarring changes, discomforts and physical weaknesses, such as: lymphedema, posture changes, sensory changes, respiratory complications, dehiscence, seroma, limitations in range of motion, loss or decrease in motor functions and pain in the homolateral limb (LEONEL; BARBOSA; MACHADO, 2017; FERREIRA; OLIVEIRA, TEIXEIRA, 2014).

All these aspects constitute complex conditions of mastectomized patients, a reality that requires specialized interventions, based on an effective care planning and Physiotherapy is an essential area of performance in postoperative situations, being able to promote a due assistance (SILVA et al., 2014).

The purpose of physiotherapeutic intervention is to provide better quality of life, when acting in the postoperative period of mastectomy can prevent and reduce complications, with guidance and early interventions and treatment of adverse effects (CERDEIRA et al., 2014).

In this sense, the study aims to investigate the role of physiotherapy in patients undergoing mastectomy.

The theme is of great relevance to the current context of health, since neoplasms appear as serious health problems and with significant incidence in women, lacking greater physiotherapeutic knowledge about their viability and effectiveness in post-mastectomy situations. It is important that the area of Physiotherapy recognizes oncology as a field of intervention and space for action, with possibilities for improvement in health, increased survival of patients affected and, above all, as a means of contributing to increasing quality of life.

METHODOLOGY

The study is based on a literature review, with searches in the Virtual Health Library (VHL) in the databases of the *Scientific Electronic Library Online (*SciELO) and Latin American and Caribbean Literature on Health Sciences (LILACS), in particular of publications in periodicals in the area of Physiotherapy.

As a search procedure, the following keywords were used in a correlated way: Physiotherapy, Post-mastectomy, Care, Treatment, Prevention.

As inclusion criteria, only scientific articles were included, from 2011-2018, complete studies, written in Portuguese and meeting the studied theme.

As exclusion criteria, we did not consider other formats of studies such as monographs, theses and dissertations, materials outside the indicated time frame, incomplete, written in other languages, not related to the theme and that deal with other types of oncological surgeries. The systematic selection of materials follows the flowchart below.

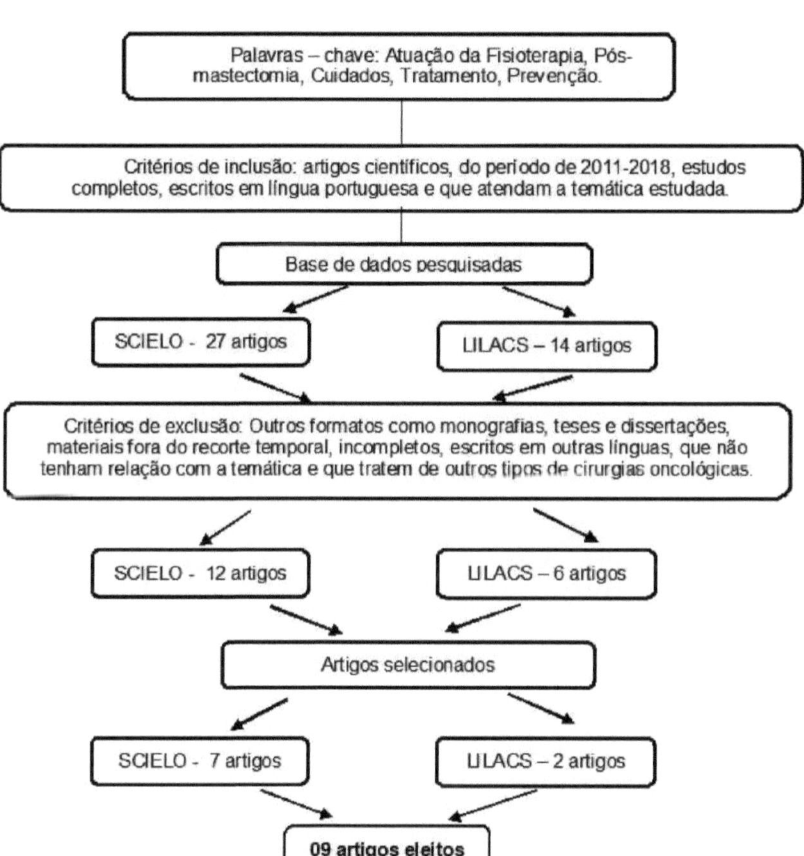

Figure 1. Flowchart of the selection of studies. Source: Prepared by the authors (June/2018)

RESULTS

The selected materials are consolidated in the synoptic table, which contains the main findings, contemplating authors, objectives, methodologies and conclusions/results of each study.

Table 1 - Consolidation of results

Authors	Objective	Methodology	Conclusion / Results
Luz and Lima (2011)	To review the literature studies in order to verify and evaluate the benefits of physiotherapeutic resources in the treatment and prevention of post-mastectomy lymphedema.	Literature review	The resources found were: complex decongestive physiotherapy; intermittent pneumatic compression; manual lymphatic drainage; compression garments; bandages; drugs; exercises; surgery; laser therapy; general care; mechanical lymphatic drainage; TENS; self-massage; hydrotherapy; microwaves; ultrasound;

			thermotherapy; balneotherapy; vertical immersion in mercury; intra-arterial injections of autologous lymphocytes; diuretics; Casley-Smith method; and high-voltage electrical stimulation (HVE). Physiotherapy, with its ample resources, is still the most efficient choice in the treatment of post-mastectomy lymphedema.
Nascimento (2012)	To investigate women after surgery for breast cancer, seeking to identify over two years the most frequent complications and the physiotherapeutic approaches most frequently adopted.	A descriptive, retrospective study, with data from 707 medical records of women operated on for breast cancer in a hospital in Campinas.	At the end of the program, most women were discharged. Over the years, there was a reduction in the frequency of shoulder range of motion restriction with increased lymphedema. Arm care, home exercises and self-drainage were the most adopted conducts.
Tacani et al. (2013)	Evaluate the effects of decongestive physiotherapy in upper limb lymphedema in patients in the late postoperative period of breast cancer	Study A retrospective study of 44 medical records of patients who underwent mastectomy	A reduction in lymphedema and of other symptoms such as pain and sensibility alterations by means of decongestive physiotherapy in the evaluated population.
Giacon et al. (2013)	To evaluate the effects of a physiotherapy protocol on range of motion and shoulder muscle strength in the postoperative period of breast cancer	Protocol for physical rehabilitation with 18 patients (divided into 2 groups) of the Liga Sorocabana de combate ao câncer (LSCC)	The results obtained in this study show that the physiotherapy treatment protocol proposed for patients in the postoperative phase of breast cancer improved the range of movement and shoulder muscle strength, however, there was no difference from the volunteers who did not receive this intervention.
Cerdeira et al. (2014)	To seek information about the role of Physiotherapy in patients after breast cancer surgery, knowing the aspects of this action.	Bibliographic review	Studies show that Physiotherapy plays a fundamental role in the prevention or reduction of possible sequels arising from the postoperative period, such as respiratory, circulatory and osteomyoarticular complications.
Silva et al. (2014)	To identify the quality of life (QoL) of mastectomized women, to relate the results to the muscular strength of the affected upper limb (ARM) and to draw a socio-functional profile.	Cross-sectional, analytical, exploratory and quantitative study with 10 women, aged 30 to 60 years, who underwent mastectomy.	The breast cancer and the mastectomy exert direct impact in the strength of MMSS, in the functionality and in the QL of women in the sexual, cognitive and emotional domains, and the physiotherapy has an important role in the rehabilitation and social reinsertion of these women.
Ferreira, Oliveira, Teixeira	To present a systematic review on the role of physiotherapy in	Systematic and descriptive	According to the studies analysed, physiotherapy in the

(2014)	the postoperative period of mastectomy and appropriate physiotherapeutic resources to be performed postoperatively.	review	postoperative period of mastectomy does not act only in the curative and rehabilitative context, but mainly in the prevention of complications and sequels of the postoperative treatment of
			mastectomy.
Souza and Souza (2014)	To highlight the importance and effectiveness of physiotherapy interventions during postoperative complications of breast cancer, showing the contribution of physiotherapy to the quality of life of these women.	Literature review	All the authors agree that the surgical removal brings harm to the movement of the limb homolateral to the surgery. Although the benefits of early functional rehabilitation in women submitted to oncologic breast surgery are widely recognized, there is no consensus as to which exercises are the most indicated, the periodicity in which they should be performed, and the duration of the program.
Leonel Barbosa and Machado (2017)	Emphasize the role of physiotherapy in the treatment of breast cancer through physiotherapeutic resources and the main complications in the postoperative period.	Literature review	The lymphedema was the main postoperative complication and kinesiotherapy was the main resource. It was verified, the important role of physiotherapy in the prevention of major complications and functional recovery of the patient after mastectomy, thus providing greater independence in daily life activities and contributing to a better quality of life.

In the quantitative nine studies that meet the research objectives were elected, being these studies mostly from the year 2014, totaling four studies, followed by two studies from the year 2013, one study from the year 2011, one corresponding to the year 2012 and one study from the period 2017.

The methodology used included 4 bibliographic reviews, 2 retrospective studies with analysis of medical records, 1 descriptive systematic review, 1 transversal analytical study with 10 patients and 1 physical rehabilitation protocol with 18 patients.

DISCUSSION

Luz and Lima (2011) evaluated that Physiotherapy based on complex decongestive therapy, manual lymphatic drainage, exercises and hydrotherapy was able to obtain more satisfactory results in the treatment of lymphedema after mastectomy surgeries. In cases of edema, however, positive results were only possible with different associated therapies such as exercises, intermittent pneumatic compression, compression garments, bandages and laser. In this context, the study of Ferreira, Oliveira, Teixeira (2014) substantiate that the protocol of kinesiotherapy and manual lymphatic drainage were the most frequent interventional therapies in cases of postoperative mastectomy, demonstrating that the range of physiotherapeutic resources promotes efficiency in treatment.

Another similar result can be observed in the research of Tacani et al (2013), who based on a retrospective study found that kinesiotherapy and decongestive Physiotherapy were techniques used that provided recovery of range of motion and functionality of the scapular girdle, as well as reduction of lymphedema, pain symptoms, scar adhesions and pericatheter sensitivity changes. In the vision of the authors, the application of the resources of Physiotherapy promoted analgesia, sensorial stimulation and increase of the extensibility of the collagen, conditions which demonstrate that the conventional techniques benefit the post mastectomized patients. However, as the authors point out, the techniques must be adapted and adequate to the patients, according to each case.

According to the study by Cerdeira (2014), Physiotherapy shows as an efficient intervention in post-mastectomy treatment, especially in lymphedema, one of the most feared complications. The physiotherapeutic action acts in the improvement of circulatory function, aiming to recover functionalities, psychological, emotional, social, and physical, seeking reinclusion of patients in everyday activities, enabling greater quality of life.

Corroborating this conception, in the research of Leonel Barbosa and Machado (2017), even considering different complications in the post-mastectomy period, such as pain, limitation of range of motion, weakness, shortening of the muscles involved in the joint of the limb homolateral to the surgery, infections, hemorrhage, edema, scar disorder, seroma, and dehiscence, there is consensus that lymphedema is the main complication in postoperative mastectomy. For the authors, physical therapy plays an important role in the prevention of these complications and in the functional recovery of patients, providing greater independence and contributing to a better quality of life.

Data correlated with these results were found in the exploratory and quantitative analytical cross-sectional study conducted by Silva et al. (2014) with 10 mastectomized women, which sought to analyze the effects of complications on functional, social and quality of life conditions. As results, it was possible to identify that the mastectomy has an impact on the muscle strength of the upper limbs, functionality and quality of life of women, in sexual, cognitive and emotional aspects. The Physiotherapy is inserted as important in the rehabilitation and social reinsertion of these women, since the physiotherapeutic action is one of the main preventive agents of complications after mastectomy.

Also in terms of prevention, the research of Ferreira, Oliveira, Teixeira (2014) reiterates that in post-operative mastectomy, Physiotherapy acts in healing and rehabilitation, but is effective mainly in preventing complications and sequelae of treatment, such as reduction of lymphedema, prevention of atrophy, adhesions, functional improvement and promoting better quality of life for patients.

In this perspective, Souza and Souza (2014), in their study on the performance of Physiotherapy in complications of postoperative breast surgery, recognize the benefits of early functional rehabilitation, however, they did not identify consensus on which exercises are most beneficial, periodicity of the intervention and the duration of the program.

The retrospective study by Nascimento (2012) investigated for two years the most frequent complications affecting mastectomized women and found that there was a reduction in the frequency of shoulder range of motion restriction with increased lymphedema. Through a rehabilitation program, the physiotherapeutic intervention was based on arm care, home exercises and self-drainage, which allowed for greater prevention, efficacy in the rehabilitation process and in the treatment of post-surgical complications. Another rehabilitation protocol was developed in the research of Giacon et al. (2013), which through physiotherapeutic treatment with groups of 18 patients allowed improvement in range of motion and shoulder muscle strength.

In the consolidated research, lymphedema appears as one of the main post-mastectomy complications and many are the physiotherapeutic resources that can be developed for the improvement of circulation, functionality and rehabilitation of movements. Prevention was highlighted as essential in postoperative complications, with contributions to improving the quality of life of patients.

CONCLUSION

The findings consist of physical therapy as a specific area of action in the prevention and recovery of post mastectomized patients, not only regarding the aspects of the disease, but especially in global rehabilitation, physical, psychological and social. Physiotherapy presents itself as an early intervention and also intervenes in the sequels, with the objective of, in the shortest time possible, enabling functional conditions for the exercise of daily activities, acting proactively in the psychosocial aspects. As a limitation of the research, it was noticed the incipiency of materials focused on partial post-mastectomy, which allows the suggestion of new studies that contemplate the performance of physical therapy with a focus on this condition.

REFERENCES

CERDEIRA, Denilson de Queiroz et al. Physical therapy in patients after breast cancer surgery: a literature review. **Revista Expressão Católica**. 2014 jan./jun.; 3(1): 23-35. Disponívelem : <http://publicacoesacademicas.fcrs.edu.br/index.php/rec/article/view/1398/113>Accessed 27 Mar. 2018.

FERREIRA, Tereza Cristina dos Reis; OLIVEIRA, Ediane da Silva Palmerim de; TEIXEIRA, Evellin dos Santos. Atuação da Fisioterapia no pósoperatório de mastectomia: revisão sistemática. **Revista da Universidade Vale do Rio Verde**, Três Corações, v. 12, n. 2, p. 765-776,aug. /dez. 2014. Disponívelem :< https://dialnet.unirioja.es/descarga/articulo/4901260.pdf.> Accessed 27 Mar. 2018.

GIACON, Fabiana Peixoto et al. Effects of physiotherapy treatment in the postoperative period of breast cancer on muscle strength and range of motion of the shoulder. **J Health Sci Inst.** 2013;31(3):316-9. Availablelem : <https://www.unip.br/presencial/comunicacao/publicacoes/ics/edicoes/2013/03_jul-set/V31_n3_2013_p316a319.pdf>.Accessed 27 Mar. 2018.

INCA. National Cancer Institute, Types of Cancer. **Estimativa 2016.** Cancer Incidence in Brazil. Available at: http://www.inca.gov.br/wcm/dncc/2015/estimativa- 2016.asp>. Accessed 10 Mar. 2018.

LEONEL, Caroline Canassa; BARBOSA, Maria Socorro dos Santos; MACHADO, Carla Komatsu. The performance of physiotherapy in the treatment of breast cancer and the main complications in the postoperative period. **Fisiosale Journal.** 2017. Available at: <http://fisiosale.com.br/assets/a-atua%C3%A7%C3%A3o-da-fisioterapia-no-tratamento-do- c%C3%A2breast-cancer-and-the-principal-complications%C3%A7%C3%B5es-no-p%C3%B3s- operat%C3%B3rio..pdf>

LUZ, Naiane Durvalina da; LIMA, Andréa Conceição Gomes. Physiotherapeutic resources in post-mastectomy lymphedema: a literature review. **Fisioter Mov**. 2011 jan/mar;24(1):191-200.Available from: <www.scielo.br/pdf/fm/v24n1/v24n1a22.pdf> Accessed 27 Mar. 2018.

NASCIMENTO, Simony Lira. Complications and physiotherapeutic conducts after surgery for breast cancer: a retrospective study. **Fisioter Pesq**. 2012; 19(3):248-255. Available at: < http://www.scielo.br/pdf/fp/v19n3/a10v19n3.pdf> Accessed on 27 Mar. 2018.

SILVA, Suelen Helena da et al. Qualidade de vida pós-mastectomia e sua relação com a força muscular de membro superior. **Fisioter Pesq.** 2014; 21(2):180-185. Disponível em:<http://www.scielo.br/pdf/fp/v21n2/pt_1809-2950-fp-21-02-00180.pdf>

SOUZA, Nathália Abdala Moitinho; SOUZA, Elsiane Stangarlin Fernandes. Atuação da fisioterapia nas complicações do pós-operatório de câncer de mama: uma revisão de literatura. Revista **UNINGÁ, Maringá** - PR, n.40, p. 175-186 abr./jun. 2014. Available at:<http://revista.uninga.br/index.php/uninga/article/download/1160/782>. Accessed on 27 Mar. 2018.

TACANI, Pascale Mutti et al. Fisioterapia descongestiva no linfedema de membros superiores pós-mastectomia: estudo retrospectivo. **Revista Brasileira de Ciências da Saúde**, ano 11, n° 37, jul/set 2013. Available at:
<http://seer.uscs.edu.br/index.php/revista_ciencias_saude/article/viewFile/1884/145>Accessed 27 Mar. 2018.

CHAPTER 4

THE ROLE OF PHYSIOTHERAPY IN THE TREATMENT OF STRESS URINARY INCONTINENCE IN WOMEN: A LITERATURE REVIEW

MARIA JOSE DA SILVA[1]

ALIDIANE BERNARDO[1]

ANDRÉA LIMA DE SÁ[2]

Urinary incontinence (UI) is any complaint about the involuntary loss of urine through the urethra, which presents itself in a negative way in the social, economic, psychological and hygienic life of the affected population. It is a public health problem found at any stage of life and in all age groups, whose risk increases with age, determining a series of consequences that can interfere with the quality of life of these people, leading them to a change in behavior, such as isolation, low self-esteem and depression, according to the International Continence Society (ICS) "*InternanationalContinenceSociety*" (BERQUÓ et al, 2009).

UI is an experience that affects millions of people of all ages, especially females. In Brazil, it is estimated that there are approximately 13 million women with different manifestations of the disease; even though there are no considerable records on the incidence and prevalence of UI. Studies in Belo Horizonte have shown that the prevalence of UI among patients admitted to nursing homes and hospitals with an average age of 72.2 years is 48.2% (BERQUÓ et al, 2016).

Several factors have been related to the occurrence of UI symptoms, the most important being: race, hormonal change, medication, obesity, alcohol, caffeine, high-impact sports, smoking, chronic cough, the advanced age, amount and type of delivery, gynaecological surgeries, the sedentary lifestyle, physical and mental disabilities and some prevalent diseases in the elderly such as stroke and Parkinson's disease, in addition to medications that are potentially capable of causing a decrease in pelvic muscle tone and/or generating nerve damage (HIGA et al, 2008; HENKES et al, 2015; TEIXEIRA et al, 2014).

With the progressive increase in the life expectancy of the population, the number of women in middle age tends to increase more and more, making UI more prevalent, which will lead to an increasing number of cases and, many of them will not be previously diagnosed due to lack of knowledge, embarrassment to talk about it or for believing that UI is a normal condition resulting from the aging process, and not a disease, leading these women to a social and family isolation, thus having their treatment neglected, worsening their condition by the delay or absence of intervention (FERNANDES et al, 2015).

Many women generally associate UI as a problem of old age that occurs due to the weakness of the body musculature that is installed as the person gets older; having these ideas already pre-established. Often these women also have other pathologies such as hypertension considered more serious and urgent, underestimating the symptom of urinary loss, believing to be a problem that does not need to be brought to the attention of a health professional, especially if this is male, because they feel embarrassed (HENKES et al, 2015).

UI can be classified in several ways, the three most common types are: stress urinary incontinence (SUI) where urinary loss occurs in situations in which there is increased intra-abdominal pressure, such as physical exercise, rapid change of posture, coughing or sneezing etc., urge incontinence (UIU) where there will occur an inability to retain urine due to a strong urinary urge and mixed urinary incontinence (MUI) is formed by the association of the two previous conditions. The most frequent among women is stress urinary incontinence (RIOS et al, 2010; BOTELHO et al, 2007).

SUI usually occurs when abdominal pressure increases, leading to extra pressure to the bladder, culminating in loss of urine. Under normal conditions the urethra is capable of withstanding any increase in abdominal pressure because the portion of the urethra, located inside the abdomen, receives the same pressure, thus neutralising the result of the effort, however, when there is a relaxation of the pelvic floor, the bladder and urethra suffer a process of herniation, so that during the effort the urethra moves to an extra-abdominal position, ceasing to receive the increase in abdominal pressure. In the absence of this compensatory increase, the bladder pressure exceeds the urethra, thus occurring urinary loss, popularly known as dropped bladder and clinically as stress urinary incontinence (OLIVEIRA et al, 2007; NASCIMENTO, 2017).

Stress Urinary Incontinence is considered a multifactorial condition that affects many people in different age groups, however the prevalence is higher in the elderly population; representing a serious public health problem, it is estimated that 45% of the female population present some type of urinary incontinence and it is calculated that 50% of these present stress urinary incontinence (SUI). This prevalence increases independently with age and parity, there are other factors that may also contribute to the worsening of the case among them are obesity, ethnicity, diabetes, ascites, hormonal changes and previous surgeries (RIOS et al, 2010; OLIVEIRA et al, 2007).

In general, SUI is multifactorial in origin and because it has a large negative impact on the quality of life of patients regardless of the type, it requires a questionnaire to assess the problem, as determined by the ICS, associated with a complete history, review of systems, tests and measures. The patient can participate actively through self-identification of the pattern of urinary symptoms in the form of notes/diary, the physiotherapist must perform an appropriate examination of the pelvic floor muscles, with internal measures of pelvic muscle strength that can be determined with special assessment instruments, such as a perineometer or digital palpation, such information forms the basis for an intervention plan (SOUSA et al, 2011).

SUI may be treated in two ways: surgical and conservative. The first is an invasive procedure, not effective in all cases and of high cost, besides the fact that symptoms recur before five years. The conservative approach, on the other hand, proposes that physiotherapy should be the first choice in the treatment of SUI due to its good results, low rate of side effects, non-invasiveness and reduced costs (MENEZES et al, 2012; SILVA et al, 2014).

Physiotherapy begins the treatment of SUI by raising awareness and giving a clear explanation about the pelvic region because most women do not know their own body, followed by behavioral therapy that helps the patient understand the need for re-education of urinary habit, guide a plan for better control of urinary desire and a hydric diet. The physiotherapeutic action consists of strengthening the pelvic floor muscles through kinesiotherapy, electrostimulation, vaginal cones and biofeedback, strategies that motivate the patient, which is essential for the success of the therapeutic approach, and an important participation both in the prevention and treatment of SUI, contributing to the rehabilitation and reintegration of the incontinent patient into society (OLIVEIRA et al, 2007; SANTOS et al, 2009).

The exercises for the pelvic floor muscles, performed with voluntary contraction that causes urethral closure, favouring continence by strengthening the perineal muscles was created in 1948, Arnold Kegel, and kinesiotherapy, which contemplates the strengthening exercises of the pelvic floor muscles, which increases the tone and urethral resistance, has determined the improvement and/or cure for more than five years in several patients (SILVA et al, 2014).

The purpose of the Biofeedback device is to provide awareness and selective control of the pelvic floor muscles and measure the action potentials of their contractions translating their intensity through visual signals, these signals increase as the contractions become more effective, informing the patient through visual or sound signals (therapist's voice command) which muscle group should be worked and therefore potentiate the effects of perineal exercises (SILVA et al, 2014).

Electro-stimulation, depending on the type of current frequency used, inhibits the detrusor muscle, thus reducing the number of urinations and consequently increasing bladder capacity. Vaginal cones can be associated with pelvic muscle exercises. It is based on stimulating the recruitment of the pubococcygeal and peripheral auxiliary muscles, which should retain the cones progressively from the lightest to the heaviest (OLIVEIRA et al, 2007).

The Physiotherapeutic approach in patients with SUI shows that it may be perfectly curable through conservative treatment, being the first option of choice for women with SUI when informed about the non-surgical and surgical alternatives. Both preoperatively, in the failures of surgical treatment or as an option of an expectation of quality of life this therapeutic modality has been the first choice alternative in the treatment of UI (OLIVEIRA et al, 2007).

The physiotherapist has an indispensable role in educating the community members, elaborating strategies to solve the problem and searching for low cost and less risky techniques, besides his qualification for the individual care of the patient (OLIVEIRA et al, 2007). Given the above, this review aims to present alternatives for physiotherapeutic treatments for SUI in women, which provide an improvement in the quality of life of the population and offer patients a minimally invasive approach.

External Female Genitalia

The external part of the female genitalia begins at the pubis to the perineum, and its structures are composed of: pubic mound, triangular prominence that lies in front of the pubic bones where it consists of adipose tissue over a layer of skin and hair to the junction of the abdominal wall; Labia majora: Are skin folds that runs from the pubic mound to the midline, above the anus, in the pudendal labia frenulum, hairs, sebaceous glands; Labia minora: has sexual function, has spongy tissue, blood vessels and glands. Medially, the labia minora have sensory nerve endings and is in continuity with the vaginal mucosa where they connect forming the foreskin of the clitoris, and subsequent form the frenulum has folds, is not hair, where the foreskin and the bridle of the clitoris, allows sexual intercourse with greater mobility (MORAIS, 2012; BARACHO, 2007).

Clitoris: is a cylindrical mass where it has corpora cavernosa, two erectile bodies, nerves and vessels; perineum: is located between the buttocks and the lower end of the trunk, the bony part of the symphysis pubis anterior, coccyx posterior and lateral ischial tuberosities, comprises the lower opening limits of the pelvis; vagina: Flattened shape, has duct that is in contact with the bladder and urethra, dorsal with the rectum and anal canal; uterine tubes: hollow structures where it has the function of capturing the egg, favorable environment for fertilization (BARACHO, 2007; OLIVEIRA et al, 2007).

The Pelvis x Pelvic Floor

It constitutes the lowest portion of the trunk and occupies an intermediate position between it and the lower limbs. It has the function of protecting the pelvic organs and consists of two iliac bones, articulated posteriorly with the sacrum and anteriorly with each other through the pubic symphysis. The iliac bone is formed by the fusion of three bones - the ilium, ischium and pubis. The walls of the pelvic cavity taper downwards like a funnel. The set of bones and muscles that occupy the base of this ring is shaped like a pelvis. The lower cavity of the pelvis connects to the pelvic floor, which is attached to the pelvic walls. The greater ischial incisure is largely filled by the piriformis muscle; it provides an exit for nerves and vessels from the pelvis to the gluteal region and the perineum (BARACHO, 2007; OLIVEIRA et al, 2007).

The unaltered bone structure and the design of the pelvic bones form two cavities: the upper, larger and shallower, corresponding to the false pelvis, which contains the abdominal organs; the lower, smaller and deeper, corresponding to the true pelvis, which houses the bladder, part of the ureters and the genital system, besides the final portion of the digestive tract, which is limited posteriorly by the sacrum and coccyx, laterally by the iliac bones and anteriorly by the pubis. In general, the female pelvis is shorter and wider than the male (BARACHO, 2007; OLIVEIRA et al, 2007).

The pelvic floor is a set of soft parts that close the pelvis and is formed by muscles, ligaments and fascia. Its functions are to support and suspend the pelvic and abdominal organs, maintaining urinary and faecal continence. The muscles of the pelvic floor also participate in the sexual function and are stretched in their maximum portion during the passage of the conceptual product. Currently, the pelvic floor is understood as the whole set of structures that give support to the abdominal and pelvic viscera. The pelvic floor consists of the coccygeal and levator ani muscles, which together are called the pelvic diaphragm (BARACHO, 2007; OLIVEIRA et al, 2007).

Urinary System

Urine is produced in the kidneys, passes through the ureters to the bladder, where it is stored and released to the exterior through the urethra. The bladder is an autonomous organ made up of smooth muscle and its function is to store urine without effort, pain and involuntary loss, and to eliminate it completely, voluntarily, without effort and also without pain. It has a storage capacity of 350 to 450 ml of urine in adults. It is located posteriorly to the symphysis pubis and anteriorly to the rectum, and in women it is also in contact with the uterus and vagina. It works as a low pressure system that accommodates increasing volumes of urine without increasing bladder pressure. The detrusor muscle in this filling phase is at rest produced by the relaxation generated by the stimulation of the beta-adrenergic sympathetic receptors which are found inside the bladder wall. Simultaneously the sympathetic stimulation of alpha adrenergic receptors present in the bladder neck and proximal urethra generates the contraction, consequently increasing the pressure. The storage function is mediated mainly by the sympathetic nervous system (BARACHO, 2007; OLIVEIRA et al, 2007).

For bladder filling to occur with low bladder pressure it is important that the detrusor muscle is not contracting and that there is an increase in urethral pressure. After filling the bladder, this mechanism becomes opposite, where the detrusor muscle contracts and the urinary sphincter relaxes, allowing its emptying to take place (OLIVEIRA, et al, 2007).

The bladder storage and emptying function depends on the interaction of the sympathetic and parasympathetic nervous systems and on the interaction of neurotransmitters, with facilitation or inhibition action of the spinal cord and higher areas of the central nervous system. The cerebellum coordinates the relaxation of the pelvic floor and also the frequency, strength and amplitude of detrusor contractions; it also interconnects with the encephalic reflex centres. The cerebral cortex exerts an inhibitory effect on urination. Urination is triggered by the peripheral nervous system and controlled by the central nervous system

(BARACHO, 2007).

Urinary Incontinence

ICS defines Urinary Incontinence as a condition in which there is an involuntary loss of urine. According to several authors, including Figueiredo (2008), UI affects around 20 to 50% of women at some stage of their lives. It is a dysfunction that causes physical, social and psychological harm, with a negative impact on quality of life.

According to Faria (2010), UI interferes with the personal life of affected women, impairs their professional performance, interferes with their sexual life, causing sexual dysfunctions and social embarrassment. Usually, incontinent women tend to isolate themselves, which leads to depression, stress, low self-esteem and feelings of shame, progressing to morbidity. The form of clinical presentation of UI is diverse and may manifest itself in three ways. These are: Stress Urinary Incontinence (SUI), Urge-incontinence (UI) also known as Overactive Bladder and Mixed Urinary Incontinence (MUI) (OLIVEIRA; GARCIA, 2011; VASCONCELOS et al, 2013).

SUI is when abdominal pressure increases, leading to extra pressure on the bladder, resulting in urine elimination. It is the most common type in the population, affecting up to 50% of incontinent women. SUI is considered to have a multifactorial etiology, affecting a large number of people, mostly women. Although it affects mainly the elderly, it may affect individuals at any stage of their lives, constituting an important public health problem. Through clinical examination and urodynamic study, the diagnosis of SUI is confirmed (FIGUEIREDO et al, 2008; BOTELHO et al, 2007; SILVA et al, 2014).

According to Oliveira and Garcia (2011), SUI is characterized by the involuntary loss of urine during effort, i.e., it occurs when it is associated with any activity that increases intra-abdominal pressure, whether through physical exercise, climbing stairs, sneezing or coughing, rapid change of positioning. It occurs due to a deficiency in the bladder and urethral support which is done by the pelvic floor muscles and/or by a weakness or lesion of the urethral sphincter.

Generally the condition is progressive, with constant leakage, in the face of ever decreasing effort. Under normal conditions the urethra is capable of withstanding any increase in abdominal pressure because the portion of the urethra, located inside the abdomen, receives the same pressure, thus neutralising the result of the effort. However, when there is a relaxation of the pelvic floor, the bladder and urethra suffer a process of herniation, so that during the effort the urethra moves to an extra abdominal position, no longer receiving the increase of abdominal pressure. In the absence of this compensatory increase, the vesical pressure (bladder) exceeds the urethral one, thus occurring urinary loss, clinically known as stress urinary incontinence. (FIGUEIREDO et al, 2008; OLIVEIRA et al, 2007)

There is a complex coordination in the organic system of the pelvic floor composed of the urinary, genital and intestinal systems, which when interrupted leads to dysfunction, with important clinical repercussions. As these three systems are intrinsically related in the function of the urinary tract and anatomical support, the basic knowledge of anatomy is essential for the propaedeutic and therapeutic evaluation of urinary incontinence. Currently, the approach to urinary incontinence requires a multidisciplinary team with the objective of improving the results of the treatment, whether clinical or surgical (BARACHO, 2007).

PHYSICAL THERAPY ACTION IN THE TREATMENT OF STRESS URINARY INCONTINENCE.

In the 1960's and 1970's great emphasis was given to surgery as the treatment of choice for urinary incontinence. More recently urologists and gynecologists have shown great interest in conservative therapies, stimulating research in the area of physiotherapy, improving the available resources and introducing new techniques that aim for a less invasive approach, with less burden, reducing the number of surgeries and providing a better quality of life for the patients. Thus, surgery has not been the first treatment option. For indication, the post-surgical benefits and risks should be considered, which should also be known by the women who will undergo the procedure (DREHER et al, 2009).

Conservative treatment has been highlighted in rehabilitation. Considering that UI is not a life-threatening condition, less aggressive treatment must be initially tried. Physiotherapy is considered to be the first-line therapy and must be indicated both for elderly patients and for those in the reproductive period, or even for those who have undergone previous unsuccessful surgical treatment, through various physiotherapeutic techniques, the most commonly used resources being pelvic floor kinesiotherapy,electrostimulation, vaginal cones, biofeedback, behavioral re-education, perianal magnetic stimulation, perineometer, (DREHER et al, 2009; SILVA et al, 2014; SANTOS et al. 2009).

At the beginning of the intervention one should opt for the evaluation of the strength of contraction and maintenance of muscle tone. This is done by evaluating the capacity to alter and/or interrupt the urine stream during urination. Incontinent patients are selected for the different modalities of treatment by simple exercises, which verify the ability to recruit the fibers of the levator ani muscle. When there are more accentuated degrees of UI patients do not respond satisfactorily to this therapeutic modality, while cases of mild and moderate SUI are easily resolved with pelvic exercises. The type of treatment to be indicated depends on the strength of the pelvic floor muscles, the ability to recognize the muscles and the degree of SUI (OLIVEIRA et al, 2007).

According to Oliveira et al. (2007), behavioural re-education promotes the re-establishment of a more frequent rhythm of urination, initially every hour, followed by a progressive increase of this interval may be of great help in the treatment of SUI. The patient is informed of the need for urinary habit re-education and instructed on strategies to control urination.

This research is justified by the large number of women who are affected by stress urinary incontinence, many of whom do not know that it is a health problem and that it can be treated through simple, non-invasive techniques and therefore often do not seek specialised help.

The well used physiotherapy techniques constitute an interesting form of treatment for these patients, as they can avoid (or at least postpone) the need for surgery or the use of drugs for the rest of their lives to regain normal continence.

This work aims to investigate through a literature review, the physiotherapeutic actions and treatment techniques that can be used in the daily conduct of women who suffer from stress urinary incontinence (SUI).

- To identify the main physical-functional alterations found in patients with stress urinary incontinence (SUI);
- To relate the main techniques and present the role of physiotherapy as the main treatment for SUI in women;
- To demonstrate which treatment method has the greatest benefits for patients;

METHODOLOGY

Characterisation of the Study

This is an exploratory study in the area of health, which addresses the topic of stress urinary incontinence, it is a literature review, which is developed from materials already prepared, consisting of books and scientific articles.

Population Sample

The sample is composed of articles and/or chapters of books collected from electronic databases, such as: the Virtual Health Library (VHL); Latin American and Caribbean Literature in Health Sciences (LILACS); International Literature in Health Sciences (MEDLINE); Regional Library of Medicine (BIREME); Scientific Electronic Library Online (Scielo); (GOOGLE ACADÊMICO) and libraries and/or personal collections of books and scientific journals. The following descriptors were used: urinary incontinence, stress urinary incontinence, physiotherapy, women's health, pelvic floor, muscle strength. As inclusion parameter we selected articles with specific publications on pathophysiology, physical therapy, physical therapy treatment of stress urinary incontinence in women, written in Portuguese and English and published in the last 10 years (2007 to 2017). Exclusion parameters: publications with dates less than 2007, articles with themes outside the proposed one, articles that approached the theme with other involved pathologies and also those that presented evaluation without interventions.

Research Procedures

It was done after analysis of the articles in accordance with the proposed subject. Soon after reading the text and producing a summary. Chapters, authors and year were selected, where all were discussed in this study and consequently inserted in the research, leading to the collection of information procedures and data presentation.

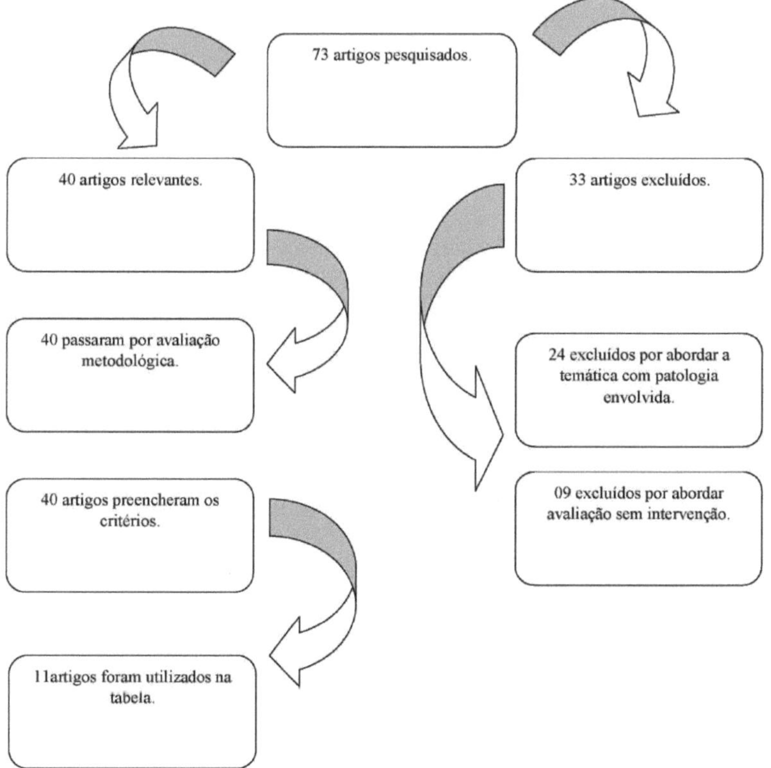

RESULTS

This study found 11 articles related to physiotherapy techniques for SUI intervention, as shown in the table below:

Figure 1 - Description of the studies on the intervention of physiotherapeutic modalities in the treatment of SUI.

Author/ Year / Journal	Type of study	Objective	Sampling	Parameters used	Main results
Golmakani et al. Oman Medical Journal (2014) Vol. 29, No. 1:32-38	Randomised clinical trial	To analyse the effectiveness of the behavioural intervention programme and vaginal cones on stress urinary incontinence.	n = 25	Use of 6 cones with similar shape and volume, numbered 1 to 6 and weighing 20, 30, 40, 50, 60 and 70 g, respectively. He was instructed to walk and not to contract his pelvic floor muscles for one minute and to check any sensation of losing the device. For three months. Questionnaires (IQOL) and (KHQ) were used for evaluation of quality of life and its improvement, After treatment.	Decreased leakage rate in the test pad was observed in both groups after 8 and 12 weeks of intervention (p <0.001, p<0.001). The intervention group was higher than in the vaginal cone group (p = 0.008). In addition, the leakage rate decreased significantly in both
Castro et al. Clinics (2008) vol.63 no.4	Controlled, single blind clinical trial,	To compare the effectiveness of pelvic floor exercises, electrical stimulation, vaginal cones and no active treatment in women with urodynamic stress urinary incontinence.	n = 27	The women were assessed before and after completion, - quality of life questionnaire (1-QOL), -pillow test, - muscle strength by the oxford scale 6-month duration	Negative pad test There was a significant decrease in the weight of the pad in all groups, - analysis between the groups, we observed that patients who used Active Treatment showed a significant decrease in the weight of the pad when compared to the control group (p = 0.003), there was no significant difference between the techniques. -I-QoL questionnaire - significant change in quality of life in comparison with the non-treated control group (p = 0.002); in relation to the techniques there was no significant improvement -MPTF group- muscular

					strength obtained significant improvement in relation to the other techniques (p = 0.002),
Santos et al. RevBrasGi necol Obstet. (2009) 31(9):447- 52	Randomised clinical trial.	To compare the effects of functional pelvic floor electrostimulation and cone therapy on women with stress urinary incontinence	n=45	- Padtest (pillow test - quality of life questionnaire - I-QoL). Micturition diary duration of treatment four monthsevaluation performed before and after treatment -GEletn groups (n=24) mean age was 55.2±12.8 sessions 20 min, 2 times per week.	There was a significant increase in quality of life - functional electrostimulation of the pelvic floor (40.3 versus 82.9) - cone therapy (47.7 versus 84.1). absorbent test, or padtest, it was observed that the same was negative, that is, the
				-GCon Group (n=21) mean age, 52.6±11.2 years, sessions of 45 min 2 times a week	The absorbent pad became "dry" in 12 (50%) and 10 (47%) of the patients treated with electrostimulation and vaginal cones, respectively. There was a significant decrease in the weight of the absorbent pad (in grams) in both groups, before and after the end of treatment (28.5 g and 32 g versus 2.0 g and 3.0 g, for EGlet and GCon, respectively) (p<0.0001).
Vural et al. Arch GynecolOb stet (2013) 288:99-103	Prospectivo controlled 0.	To evaluate the effective Sensitivity of the use of vaginal docone in patients with Stress Urinary Incontinence.	n = 22	Vaginal taping consisted of a 40 minute, daily session over a period of 12 weeks in the resting position, and to push back the vaginal taper if they felt they slipped for 15 times. 1-h padtest were performed at the beginning and after 2 months of treatment.	Vaginal cone can be treatment done in clinic or at home. 1-h padtest before and after treatment for cone group were 16.32 ± 25.70 and 0.89 ± 2.13 g, In vaginal cone group, statistically significant differences Comparison with baseline was observed in mean.
Aksaca et al.Gynecol ObstetInve st (2013) 56:23-27	Randomized, controlled, prospective	Pelvic floor muscle biofeedback for the treatment of stress urinary incontinence.	n = 20	Patients were evaluated via pad test, perineometry, pelvic floor muscle strength based on digital palpation 8 weeks after treatment. All sessions lasted 20 minutes of 40 cycles with 10 s of	Biofeedback with the best result of pelvic floor muscle strength compared to digital palpation. Padtest revealed 75% cure and 25% Improvement in the digital palpation group.

				activity followed by 20 s of relaxation.	
Lee at al. The Internationa 1 Urogynecol ogical Association (2013)	Randomi zado.	To compare the effects of pelvic floor muscle training with and without biofeedback on stress urinary incontinence.	n = 56	Padtest was used to evaluate biofeedback intervention, 12 weeks. 0 quality of life questionnaire was performed at baseline and after 4 and 12 weeks of treatment. ■	Pelvic floor muscle training using biofeedback can be conservative effective and safe, in a test pad it decreased significantly from 20.6 ± 20.0 g to 7.3 ± 13.6 g after intervention.
Hirakawa et al. The Internationa l Urogynecol ogical Association (2013)	Randomi zado.	Hypothesis To compare the effects of pelvic floor muscle training, biofeedback for stress urinary incontinence.	n = 23	Women in the BF group confirmed visit to the physiotherapist at 2, 4, 8e 12 weeks, Pelvic floor muscle contraction was checked by palpation of the perineal body, QOL was assessed by Questionnaire The primary and secondary outcome measures were assessed before and after the 12 weeks of physical training.	In both groups, there were no significant differences between groups in the changes in any of the parameters assessed.
Castro et al. Clinics (2008) vol.63 no.4	Controlled, single blind clinical trial,	To compare the effectiveness of pelvic floor exercises, electrical stimulation, vaginal cones and no active treatment in women with urodynamic stress urinary incontinence.	n = 27	The women were evaluated before and after completion, - quality of life questionnaire (I-QOL), -pillow test, -muscle strength by the oxford scale, -6-month duration	-Negative cushion test There was a significant decrease in cushion weight in all groups, analysis between groups, we observed that patients who used active treatment showed a significant decrease in cushion weight compared to the control group (p = 0.003), between techniques there was no significant difference
					- I-QoL questionnaire- significant change in quality of life compared to the untreated controls group (p = 0.002); in relation to the techniques there was no significant improvement -muscle strength PFMT-group obtained significant improvement in relation to the other techniques (p = 0.002),
Silva et al.	This is a	To evaluate the	n= 6	Age range: 51 to 73	Quality of life

Journal of Amazon Health Science (2015) Vol.1, n.1	field study where data collection was carried out in loco.	possible benefits of the exercise programme and its impacts on quality of life.		years (61 3 ± 5.63). The exercises lasted for 9 weeks, once a week, for 30 minutes.	questionnaire Total score initial 80.2+12.5 final 82.2+16.3.
Ferreira et al. revportsaúd e (2012) 30(1):3-10	Experientia l study.	To compare the influence of pelvic floor muscle training programmes with supervision and at home with the pelvic floor muscle training programme at home, on the quality of life of women with stress urinary incontinence.	n= 34	Duration of 45min twice a week; evaluation in two times at the beginning and at the end of treatment, quality of life and frequency of UI episode were evaluated Age 50.7 ± 9.3 53.9 ± 8.7	Group EG - QL (initial and final) 2.5 ± 0.8 1.7 ± 0.8 Group CG- QL (initial and final) 2.5 ± 0.8 1.7 ± 0.8 p= 0.022* 0.628(initial and final) Comparison of the frequency of incontinence episodes between groups: EG -Initial evaluation - 11.3 ± 7.2 - Final evaluation (6th month) 4.5 ± 5.1 CG - Initial assessment 11.3 ± 5.7 - Final assessment (6th month) 6.4 ± 7.5.
Sousa et al. Fisioter Mov. (2011) 24(1):39-46	study, of the experime ntal type.	To evaluate pelvic floor muscle strength and quality of life in women with complaints of urinary incontinence after kinesiotherapy.	n=22	-Functional assessment of the pelvic floor musculature (PFM); -evaluate the contraction pressure exerted by the pelvic floor musculature by perineometer -evaluate the quality of life using the King's Health questionnaire (KHQ), duration of exercise twice a week, individually, with an average duration of 30min total 12 sessions. Age (years) 65,644.09	Pre and post treatment result: AFA:1.35±0.92 3.78 ± 0.51* contraction pressure: Peak: 0.44 ± 0.30 1.0 ± 0.44*. time: 1.65 ± 1.15 4.43 ± 1.03* (significant result between pre and post treatment (p *í* 0.001)). quality of life questionnaire: Total 28.9 ± 24.3 16.8 ± 20.5
Zanetti et al. Sao Paulo Med. J. (2007) vol.125 no.5	Randomize d, prospective and controlled study.	To compare the results of the treatment of female stress urinary incontinence with pelvic floor muscle exercises with or without the supervision of a physiotherapist	n= 44	-Group A: supervised perineal exercises-23 patients who performed perineal exercises under the guidance of a physiotherapist (twice a week for 45 minutes). -Group B: unsupervised perineal exercises (control group)-21 patients who performed perineal exercises at home with	After 3 months of treatment a significant difference was observed: I-Qol - before and after treatment (82 - 79 points), p=0.2731 (control group) versus (6989 points), p=0.0001 (intervention group), Padtest :before and after treatment (24.7-15 g) p=0.0475 (control group) versus (20.1 - 3.2 g) p=0.0002 (intervention

				monthly evaluation by a physiotherapist, age between 54 and 56 years, evaluated by I-Qol, padtest	group)
Silva et al. Journal of Amazon Health Science (2015) Vol.1, n.1	Experiential study.	Verify the effectiveness of the pelvic floor muscle rehabilitation (PFMRP) in female volleyball athletes,	n=32	Evaluation of the daily micturition pillow test.	Pad test variation: -EG (n = 16) (-) 2 ± 1.28;p<0.001 * (amount of urine leakage decreased in 45.5% of athletes under PFMRP intervention) CG (n = 16) (-) 0.2 ± 0.41; p=0.324 (amount of urine leakage decreased 4.9% of athletes in CG). with statistical differences between groups (p <0.001). reduction in leakage frequency:14.3% in EG and 0.05% in CG, statistically significant difference between groups (p <0.001).

QL comparison

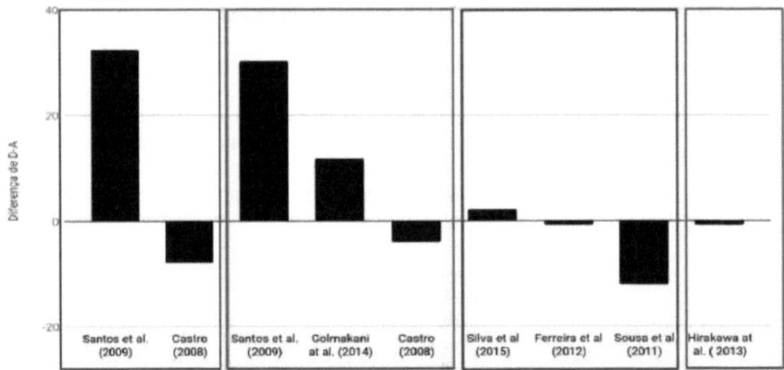

Graph 1: Represents the difference between the mean values (after minus before) of the Quality of Life Questionnaire after the respective physiotherapeutic techniques; black box Electrostimulation; red Cones; blue Kinesiotherapy; green Biofeedback

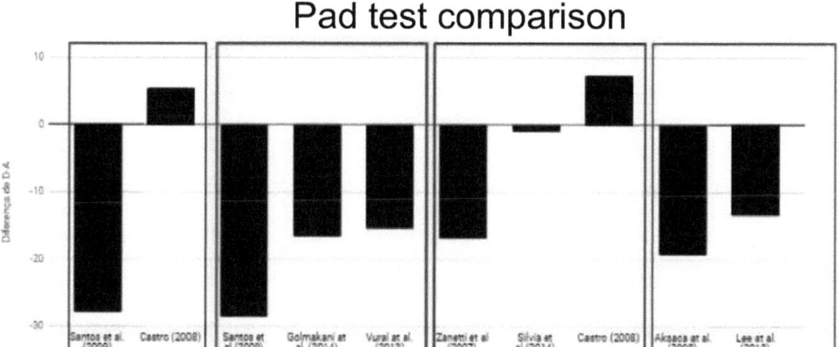

Graph 2: Represents the difference between the average values (after minus before) of the Pad Test Questionnaire after the respective physiotherapy techniques black frame Electrostimulation; red Cones; blue Kinesiotherapy; green Biofeedback

DISCUSSION

SUI is the most common type in the population, affecting up to 50% of incontinent women; it is considered to have a multifactorial etiology, affecting a large number of people, mostly women. Although it affects mainly the elderly, it may also affect individuals at any stage of their lives, constituting a public health problem. (FIGUEIREDO et al, 2008; BOTELHO et al, 2007; SILVA et al, 2014).

According to Oliveira and Garcia (2011), SUI is characterized by the involuntary loss of urine during exertion such as: physical exercise, climbing stairs, sneezing or coughing, rapid change of position. This has a negative impact on the quality of life of patients.

Due to the many factors involved in the cause of female urinary incontinence, different clinical and surgical treatments have emerged. Aiming to provide the patient with an efficient, low invasive, low cost treatment that reduces and/or eliminates the discomfort caused by urinary loss, the physiotherapeutic techniques constitute therapy capable of treating this disease by improving the muscular and nervous structures of the pelvic organ support apparatus (SARTORI, 2011).

Before proposing any treatment technique, it is important to carry out a complete assessment, with a questionnaire to evaluate the problem (quality of life questionnaire), as determined by the ICS, associated with a complete history containing identification data, anamnesis and physical examination, review of systems, tests and measures.

The patient can actively participate through self-identification of the pattern of urinary symptoms in the form of notes/diary, the physiotherapist must perform adequate examination of the pelvic floor muscles, with internal measures of pelvic muscle strength always observing the integrity, perception capacity, coordination of contraction, as well as relaxation of the structures, using evaluative techniques already validated and recommended in the literature and clinical practice that can be determined with special evaluation instruments, such as a perineometer device or digital palpation (FITZ et al. 2012; RETT et al, 2007).

The main muscle strength assessment scales described are: Pelvic Floor Functional Assessment, Oxford Scale, pad test, Quality of life questionnaire (I-Qol). Such information forms the basis for an intervention plan. Several forms of assessment and treatment are described in the literature, however, there is little consensus on which would be the most appropriate and standardized for the Pelvic Floor and adjacent structures (SOUSA et al, 2011;GOLMAKANI et al, 2014).

In the present study, a pad test and the I-Qol were used. The pad test consists of placing a pad, i.e. an absorbent, whose weight is previously measured on a precision scale and then asks the patient to perform stress manoeuvres, after which the pad is removed and her weight is measured again, the difference in weights characterises the loss of urine, fluctuations in weight greater than one gram are considered urinary incontinence (GOLMAKANI et al, 2014; SATORI, 2011).

The IQOL (IncontinenceQualityofLife) questionnaire is a specific instrument for patients with urinary incontinence. It was elaborated with the objective of reflecting the impact on the daily life of people with urinary incontinence and to be used in epidemiological studies. This study addressed the quality of life of incontinent women, this being the instrument used to assess these women undergoing physiotherapy treatment (GOLMAKANI et al, 2014).

One of the main objectives of physiotherapy treatment is to increase the resistance of the urethra and re-establish the function of the structures that support the pelvic organs. Therefore, the aim is to strengthen the pelvic floor muscles, because the improvement of the strength and function of these muscles favours a conscious and effective contraction, thus avoiding urinary loss. The main techniques used are: Kinesiotherapy, Electrostimulation, vaginal cones and Biofeedback (SILVA et al, 2015; SOUZA et al, 20011; SANTOS et al, 2009; FITZ et al, 2012; GOLMAKANI et al, 2014).

Kinesiotherapy for pelvic floor muscle training is considered a first line treatment for dysfunctions related to urinary incontinence, since it promotes an increase in PFM strength and resistance, generating an improvement in incontinence pictures. This occurs because when performing PFM training, the urethral closure force will be enough to maintain the continence mechanism at the moment when the intra-abdominal pressure increases, i.e. during coughing or physical exercise; however, in order to obtain a satisfactory result, active participation, a good understanding and acceptance on the part of patients are necessary, obeying the protocol prescribed by the physiotherapist (SILVA, et al, 2014).

As shown by Silva et al, (2015) in their study, after the evaluations, patients underwent 2 protocols: first prevention protocol composed of Kegel exercises, applied once a week for 09 weeks, totaling 09 sessions lasting 30min. After pelvic floor awareness and mobilization of the hip, the perineal exercises were performed. Starting with 4 series of 4 contractions, with an 8-second interval between each series, contracting hard and fast, the elderly being guided to contract and relax the pelvic floor muscles, thus working the type II fibers (fast contraction) (SILVA et al, 2015).

In phase 2, 4 series of 4 contractions were performed, with a 4-second interval between each contraction, the guidelines were to contract the pelvic floor muscles as hard as possible, and maintain the contraction for 2 seconds and relaxing for 2 seconds, work directed towards the type I fibres (slow contraction) (SILVA et al,

2015).

At the end, the participants were submitted to re-evaluation, using the same procedure of the evaluation form and initial questionnaire. Even presenting a positive response, the results obtained with the quality of life questionnaire were not significant (p=0.73) (SILVA et al, 2015).

There are still controversies in the literature regarding the isolated applicability of pelvic kinesiotherapy in relation to its association with electrostimulation. Beuttenmuller et al. (2011) conducted a study with 80 women with SUI, in order to compare the improvement of pelvic floor function after pelvic kinesiotherapy associated or not with electrostimulation. In their results there was no significant difference between the groups, concluding that pelvic kinesiotherapy alone or associated with electrostimulation showed the same result. (SOUZA et al. 20011; SILVA et al, 2015).

Electrostimulation provides passive strengthening of PFM and improves the perception of these muscles, stimulating the correct contraction of slow twitch fibers and fast twitch fibers and makes it possible to determine the region of the muscles or the muscle to be stimulated as for example the levator ani muscle states Castro et al, (2008). Depending on the frequency, contraction time and rest, it is possible to determine which types of fibres will be worked. Activating fast twitch fibres, during situations of increased abdominal pressure, these fibres contract quickly and reflexively preventing urinary loss.

Electrical stimulation results in inhibition of the urination reflex, as it keeps the bladder at rest, triggering an improvement in storage capacity and reducing micturition frequency, this happens because the afferent fibres of the pudendal nerve are activated, thus the pudendal nerve activates the efferent fibres of the hypogastric nerve, triggering detrusor relaxation, simultaneously, the pudendal nerve inhibits the pelvic nerve, responsible for detrusor contraction (CASTRO et al, 2008)

Functional electrostimulation of the pelvic floor and cone therapy in women with stress urinary incontinence (SUI). Randomized clinical trial with 24 women (voiding diary, padtest and quality of life questionnaire, two weekly sessions lasting 20 minutes each for four months). Method 10cm long and 3.5 cm wide, positioned in the middle third of the vagina current intensity varying from 10 to 100 mA and frequency fixed at 50. The cones from 20 to 100 g. after treatment was obtained a significant decrease in the number of urinary losses (SANTOS et al, 2009).

Biofeedback provides a better way to demonstrate the control of MAP and quantify the contraction of these muscles through action potential signals, visual signals making it possible to increase contractions enabling the patient to have a visual perception, sound, verbal command of the therapist, thus enhancing the effects of perineal exercises (SILVA et al, 2014).

To analyze the effect of adding biofeedback (BF) to the training of the pelvic floor muscles SUI. 40 women were chosen 40 and 16 participated in the conduct, starting with three series of ten slow contractions, the maintenance time of six to eight seconds in each contraction, rest six to eight and then three to four fast contractions totaling 12 sessions. Resulting in a decrease in urinary loss, improving MAP function, reduction of urinary symptoms, and a good quality of life (FITZ et al., 2012).

Efficacy of a vaginal cone program intervention in stress urinary incontinence. 60 women aged 25-65, however only 30 used vaginal cones, 30 the behavioural intervention group were instructed on pelvic floor exercise and bladder control strategies. For 12 weeks and followed up every 2 weeks (FITZ et al,2012).

Santos et al., (2009), applied two protocols in the treatment of UI, one group with electrostimulation and the other with vaginal cones, both under the supervision of a physiotherapist. The two techniques were effective in treating women with SUI. Vaginal cones, for example, stimulated the recruitment of type I and type II fibres, improving proprioception of the pelvic muscles and promoting an increase in muscle strength. Vaginal cones and behavioural education programmes are methods that give good treatment results for mild to moderate SUI, but the behavioural intervention programme is superior to vaginal cones in terms of cost, effectiveness and effects (GOLMAKANI et al, 2014).

It is an effective method for the rehabilitation of the pelvic floor muscles having as an advantage easy handling, portable, has several weights and allows an increase in muscle tone. Using a set of cones of equal sizes, but increasing weight, introduced into the vagina where the patient has to contract to hold it, provides an internal physiotherapy that quickly restores muscle tone, defines Golmakani et al, 2014.

Chart 1, Santos et al, (2009) and other authors show that in the quality of life questionnaire, the studies showed positive results for electrostimulation techniques, vaginal cones and kinesiotherapy; the other studies did not show significant results.

Graph 2, the pad test (Padtest), the results found by the authors were very significant in relation to the daily change of pads, where they present the electrostimulation, vaginal cones, kinesiotherapy and biofeedback as the best resources for the treatment of the discomfort of urinary loss.

Other methods of interventions such as electroacupuncture, magnetic stimulation and endovaginal electrostimulation are described in the literature as efficient and non-invasive techniques proposed in the treatment of stress urinary incontinence, but there was not enough material found to be presented in the present study.

There are many studies described on the subject addressed, however, few have scientific relevance, since there is no standardization of research, lack of consensus on evaluation criteria, the characteristics of the very divergent samples, and the intervention protocols are not well defined, thus limiting the research. Another limitation of the current study is the lack of follow-up to attest if the improvements achieved with the different techniques will last in the long term. In view of the above, it is necessary to develop rules for future research to have a more reliable character.

CONCLUSION

Physiotherapy in the treatment of SUI is effective, both in reducing urinary loss and improving the quality of life of incontinent women, regardless of the resource applied, as presented in the study, Kinesiotherapy, electrostimulation, vaginal cones and Biofeedback are effective treatment strategies in the therapy of SUI. These procedures are easy to apply, low cost and without side effects, providing benefits to the population, and can be used in the prevention and treatment of this pathology.

This review suggests that physiotherapy through pelvic floor muscle training should be the first line treatment for stress urinary incontinence and the physiotherapeutic techniques (kinesiotherapy, biofeedback, vaginal cones and electrostimulation) are especially indicated especially when women cannot voluntarily contract the pelvic floor muscles.

REFERENCES

AKSACA,B; etal. **BiofeedbackandPelvicFloorExercisesfortheRehabilitationofUrinaryStressIncontinence** - GynecolObstetInvest 2003;56:23-27 DOI: 10.1159/000072327

BARACHO, E. **Fisioterapia aplicada á Obstetrícia, Uroginecologia e Aspectos de Mastologia**. 4. ed Rio de Janeiro: Guanabara Koogan, 2007

BERQUÓ, M S; RIBEIRO, MO; AMARAL, RG. **Fisioterapia No Tratamento Da Incontinência Urinaria Feminina-Revisão,**Femina , July 2009 , Vol 37, N° 7.

BEUTTENMULLER, Let al. **Contração Muscular do Assoalho Pélvico De Mulheres Com Incontinência Urinária de Esforço Submitted to Exercises and Electrotherapy: Um Estudo Randomizado-** Fisioterapia e Pesquisa, São Paulo, v.18, n.3, p. 210-6 ,jul/set. 2011. BERQUÓ,MS; RIBEIRO,MO; AMARAL,RG. **Qualidade De Vida De Mulheres Portadoras De Incontinência Urinária Antes E Depois A Fisioterapia Realizada No Hospital Materno Infantil De Goiânia Goiás** - - RevCien Escol EstadSaudPubl Cândido Santiago RESAP. 2016;2(2):104-122 ISSN: 24473406

BOTELHO, F; SILVA, C; CRUZ, F. **Incontinencia Urinaria Feminina** -- ActoUrulogica 2007, 24;l 79-82

CASTRO, RAetal.**Single-blind, Randomized, CcontrolledTrialofPelvicFloorMuscle Training, ElectricalEtimulation, Vaginal Cones, and no Active Treatment in theManagement of stress UrinaryIncontinence-** Clinics2008;64:

465-72-
http://dx.doi.org/10.1590/S1807-59322008000400009

DREHER, DZ et al. **Pelvic Floor Strengthening with Vaginal Cones: A Home Care Program**, Scientia Medica, Porto Alegre, v. 19, n. 1, p. 43-49, Jan/Mar. 2009

FARIAS,CA; et al.**Impact of the type of urinary incontinence on the quality of life of female users of the Unified Health System in Southeastern Brazil -** RevBrasGinecol Obstet. 2015; 37(8):374-80

FERNANDES, S; et al. **Quality of Life in Women with Urinary Incontinence**, Revista De Enfermagem Referencia Serie Iv-N°5-.2015

FERREIRA, M; Santos PC. **Impact of training programs on the quality of life of women with stress urinary incontinence** - Rev. Port. Saúde Pública. 2012;30(1):3- 10

FERREIRA, S; et al. **Reeducationofpelvicfloormuscles in volleyballathletes** - RevAssocMedBras 2014; 60(5):428-433

FIGUEIREDO, EM; et al. **Perfil SociodemográfiCo E Clinico De Usuárias De Serviço De Fisioterapia Uroginecológica Da Rede Pública** - RevBrasFisioter. 2008;12(2):136-42.

FITZ ,FF; et al. **Effect of adding biofeedbackaotraining of the floor muscles**

pelvic for the treatment of stress urinary incontinence - RevBrasGinecol Obstet. 2012; 34(11):505-10

GOMES, GV;SILVA,G D. **Incontinencia Urinaria De Esforço Em Mulheres Pertencentes Ao Programa De Saúde Da Familia De Dourados** (MS), Rev. AssocMedBras 2010.

GOLMAKANI, N; et al **BehavioralInterventionProgram versus Vaginal Cones on Stress**

UrinaryIncontinenceandRelatedQualityofLife: A RandomizedClinicalTrial - Oman Medical Journal (2014) Vol. 29, No. 1:32-38 DOI 10. 5001/omj.2014.08

HIGA, R; et al. **Experiences of Brazilian Women with Urinary Incontinence.**Texto Contexto Enferm, Florianópolis, 2010 Oct-Dec; 19(4): 627-35.

HIGA, R; LOPES, M H B M; REIS, M J. **Fatores De Risco Para Incontinência Urinária Na Mulher.** RevEscEnferm USP 2008; 42(1):187-92. www.ee.usp.br/reeusp/ 187

HIRAKAWA,R; et al. **RandomizedControlledTrialOfPelvicFloorMuscle Training WithOrWithoutBiofeedbackForUrinaryIncontinence -** IntUrogynecol J DOI 10.1007/s00192-012-2012-8

HENKES, DF; et al. **Urinary incontinence: the impact on the life of affected women and the meaning of physiotherapeutic treatment**. Semina: Biological and Health Sciences, Londrina, v. 36, n. 2, p. 45-56, jul./dez. 2015.

LEE, HN; etal . **PelvicFloorMuscleTraining UsingAnExtracorporealBiofeedbackDeviceFor Female Stress UrinaryIncontinence -** IntUrogynecol J (2013) 24:831-838 DOI 10.1007/s00192-012-1943-4

PINHEITO, BF; et al. **Physiotherapy for Perineal Consciousness: A Comparison Between Kinesiotherapies With Digital Touch and Biofeedback -** Fisioter. Mov., Curitiba, v. 25, n. 3, p. 639-648, Jul/Sep. 2012

MENEZES, G M D; et al.**Queixa De Perda Urinária**: **um problema silente pelas mulheres**. - RevGaúchaEnferm, Porto Alegre (RS) 2012 mar;33(1):100-8

MORAIS, PINTO JAIME ANTONIA. **Evolução Eletromiografia Do Assoalho Pelvico Com a Utilização Da Eletroestimulação Na Incontinência Urinária De Esforço:** Trabalho de Conclusão de curso, extremo sul catarinense, 2012.

NASCIMENTO, SIMONE MATTOS. **Avaliação Fisioterapeutica Da Força Muscular do Assoalho Pelvico Na Mulher Com Incontinencia Urinaria de Esforço após Cirurgia de Wertheim-Meigs:** Revisão, Revista Brasileira De Cancerologia 2009.

OLIVEIRA,JR; GARCIA,RR. **Cinesiotherapy in the treatment of urinary incontinence in elderly women,** Rev. Bras. Geriatr. Gerontol, Rio De Janeiro, 2011; 14(2):343-351

OLIVEIRA,KAC; RODRIGUES, ABC; PAULA, AB. **TecinicasFisiterapeuticas No Tratamento E Prevenção Da Incontinencia Urinaria De Esforço Na Mulher**. Article Published in the electronic journal F@Pciencia, Apucarana-Pr, V.1, N°1, 31-40, 2007

RIOS,J L;SILVA, BA. **Pathophysiology of stress urinary incontinence. Review article** - http://www.efdeportes.com/ Revista Digital - Buenos Aires - Year 14 - No 140 - January 2010

RETT, M. T. et al.**Quality of life in women after treatment for incontinence urinária de esforço com fisioterapia.** Revista Brasileira de Ginecologia e Obstetrícia. Vol. 29. N. 3, 2007

SANTOS,PFD; et al. **Functional electrostimulation of the pelvic floor versus therapy with vaginal cones for the treatment of stress urinary incontinence** - - RevBrasGinecol Obstet. 2009; 31(9):447-52

SILVA, GC.; FREITAS,AO.; SCARPELINI, P.; HADDAD, CAS. **Tratamento Fisioterapeutico Da Incontinência Urinaria De Esforço - Relato De Caso**, RevistaUnilus Ensino E Pesquisa - Vol. 11, N° 25 , Ano 2014

SILVA, REG; et al. **Kinesiotherapeutic Treatment as a Measure for the Prevention of Stress Urinary Incontinence in Elderly Women and its Relation to the Quality Of Life -** JournalofAmazon Health Science Vol.1, n.1, 2015.

SOUSA, JG. *et al.* **Evaluation of Pelvic Floor Muscle Strength in Elderly Women with Urinary Incontinence.** Fisioterapia em Movimento. Vol. 24. N. 1, 2011.

SARTORI, D. V. B. **Effect of Electrostimulation and Perineal Exercises in Women with Stress Urinary Incontinence.** Essays and Science: Biological, Agricultural and Food Sciences Saúde. Vol. 15. N. 4, 2011

TEIXEIRA, C.; NOGUEIRA, P.; MASCARENHAS T. **Tratamento Da Incontinência Urinaria De Esforço,** Review article, Acta ObstetGinecolPort 2014.

VASCONCELOS, CTM; et al. **Pelvic floor dysfunctions: sociodemographic and clinical profile of users of an urogynecology outpatient clinic -** Revista Eletrônica Gestão & Saúde ISSN:1982-4785

VEY, APZ; et al. **Female Stress Urinary Incontinence: Evaluation and Proposal of Physiotherapeutic Treatment-** Biomotriz, v.10, n. 01, p. 24 - 39, jul./2016 24

VURAL, M; et al. **Vaginal Cone Therapy In PatientsWith Stress UrinaryIncontinence** - ArchGynecolObstet (2013) 288:99-103DOI 10.1007/s00404-012-2701

ZANETTE, MRD; et al. **ImpactOfSupervisedPhysiotherapeuticPelvicFloorExercises For TreatingFemale Stress UrinaryIncontinence -** Sao Paulo Med. J. vol.125 no.5 São Paulo Sept. 2007

CHAPTER 5

PHYSIOTHERAPIST INTERVENTION AFTER CHILDBIRTH: DIASTASIS TREATMENT

CHEYLA OLIVEIRA VIEIRA[1]
WILMA LEÔNCIO CHACON[15]

The study highlights an analysis of the physiotherapist's intervention in the postpartum period. Stage resulting from hormonal changes that interfere in the circulatory, respiratory, urinary, nervous, digestive and skeletal muscle systems. However, these changes need to be accompanied to help women return to their natural state after giving birth (TALLAH; TREVISANI, 20150).

Women build their life project from a very early age, that is, to grow up, find a loving partner and from there build a family. Influenced by several types of motivations, which will give origin to the desire of having a child. This moment requires physical and psychological preparation, as a way to bring positive results for pregnancy until delivery (STEPHENSON, et al.,2008).

During pregnancy, when going into labor, there is the action of processes that act inside the uterus in order to expel the fetus through contractile activity. However, the pain during this moment is unique to each woman, which can be influenced by various factors, i.e. cultural aspect, anxiety and fear (ANDRADE, et al., 2011).

Childbirth can be defined as the resolving stage of the puerperal pregnancy cycle, where pregnancy corresponds to the evolution and the puerperium a mechanical event.In addition to the process marked by changes that the woman goes through, uterine growth causes the stretching of abdominal muscles in the formation of diastasis. Characterized as space between the muscle from the upper abdomen to below the navel.According to Garcia (2007).

The formation of diastasis does not usually trigger pain or discomfort for the woman, being seen as a process that acts slowly. However, it is more evident in women who do not have a good abdominal tonus before becoming pregnant. During this stage, there is an increase in the ultra-abdominal pressure causing the uterus to be pushed outward, assisting in the passage of the fetus.

Several studies have been conducted on assistance to women during pregnancy and labor because of complications for both mother and baby. In this way, facing adversities in maternal health care has involved initiatives from various organs and organizations of governmental or non-governmental aspects as a way of reducing statistics.According to Janine Schirmer (2000).

During pregnancy it is even more important to take care not only of the baby's good development, but also of the pregnant woman's body. Regular prenatal care and a balanced and healthy diet help reduce body changes. Among the alterations, the increase in lumbar and thoracic curvatures can be highlighted. After delivery, these deviations remain and need to be treated by the physiotherapist.Silva et al., (2010).

Gentle exercises can be performed postpartum to strengthen the tone and increase the support functions of the abdominal muscles. Among the benefits are the re-education and strengthening of the abdominal muscles, correction of posture, physical conditioning and relaxation; even causing comfort to the woman.(BARACHO, 2007).

Before starting the activities it is essential that the woman undergoes an assessment. In this way, she will be sure of the type of exercise she can do and the possible risks. The physiotherapist will prescribe an exercise program, guide on the posture, in the proposed treatment of diastasis of the rectus abdominis muscles so common among women, resulting from childbirth (KISNER; COLBY, 2010).

When analyzing the studies previously published on the treatment of abdominal diastasis in the postpartum period under the physiotherapeutic aspect, it is necessary to highlight some theorists who contributed to the theme, such as: Andrade et al., (2011), Baracho (2012), Garcia (2007), Mesquita et al., (2015), Polden; Mantle (2017) Silva (2010), among others who added positively.

The methodology is characterized by an integrative review of qualitative and quantitative aspect through scientific articles published in the Scielo, Lilacs, Medline databases between 2010 and 2017. It is necessary to update information on the subject in question, bringing new perspectives and directions regarding the treatment of diastasis and the role of the physiotherapist. The research presents as a question: Can abdominal diastasis be treated through a physiotherapeutic perspective?

The theme about the importance of physiotherapy in the postpartum period is justified in order to arouse new studies, to think of alternatives that encourage the work of the physiotherapist and resources used to patients in the treatment of diastasis. In order to support the development of public health policies, focusing on the monitoring of women after childbirth by a team with different views of assistance. Considering that during the puerperium, characterised by the variable chronological period in which changes occur in the anatomy and physiology of women (MANTLE; POLDEN, 2010). The relevance of this process is proportional to the gestational transformations during pregnancy. By rule, the authors emphasize that the puerperal involution happens within 6 weeks, although it is important to understand the period that happens at delivery.

This article aims to understand the role of physiotherapy and the different treatments and as specific objective: Understand the physical and physiological changes in pregnancy; Characterize the diaphragmatic breathing exercise associated with the perineum; Highlight its benefits in diastasis.

METHODOLOGY

Study design

The integrative review corresponds to a research method used that involves the systematization and publication of the results of the literature search so that they can be useful in health care. The integrative review includes the analysis of relevant research that provides support for decision-making and improvement of the clinical aspect, enabling the understanding of the study Galvão et al (2008).

The method aims to gather and systematize research results on a limited topic in an orderly manner, contributing to the knowledge of the investigated topic. For Tallah, Trevisani (2015), the studies included in the review are analyzed systematically in relation to their objectives, materials and methods, allowing the reader to analyze the pre-existing knowledge on the investigated theme.

The qualitative aspect has the purpose of understanding the phenomena it studies and the actions that will be performed by the researcher (GIL, 2012). Based on the perspective of individuals who participate in the situation or aspect of the research. Without worrying about the numerical or quantitative representativeness of the data highlighted, statistics and cause and effect relationships as happen in the quantitative approach.

During the investigation, it is necessary to recognize the complexity of the object of study, review the theme, establish concepts, analyze theories, use data collection techniques and, finally, evaluate all the material in a specific and contextualized way (FONSECA, 2010). Qualitative research works with the constructed universe of meanings, corresponding to processes and phenomena that cannot be reduced to the operationalization of variables.

For the content analysis, the researcher gathers the collected data and after organizing the material, he/she goes to the step of categorizing the information (BAUER, 2012). The data categorization corresponds to the main moment of the research, which consists in the separation of excerpts of the texts into categories based on the theoretical framework and information analysis.

The quantitative nature takes into account the determination of the composition and sample size as fundamental principles in the representation of statistical data, according to Lakatos; Marconi (2010). It seeks the validation of hypotheses based on structured and numerically described data, quantifying and generalizing the results.

With regard to the articles used in the study, they were based on the theoretical structure produced nationally as the development of the keywords: diastasis of the rectus abdominis muscles, treatment, physiotherapy, postpartum stage. In which prioritized as steps: separation of articles, identification of the theme, reading the titles, abstracts of the studies previously built and preparation of the research;

considering the inclusion and exclusion criteria.

Sample population

The methodology is characterized by a qualitative and quantitative integrative review on the role of the physiotherapist in the treatment of diastasis of the rectus abdominis muscles during the months of April to November 2017 through the database of the Scientific Electronic Library Online (SCIELO), Latin American and Caribbean Literature on Health Sciences (LILACS) and International Literature in Health Sciences (MEDLINE) in Portuguese language.

Inclusion and exclusion criteria

Articles that presented studies on diastasis of the rectus abdominis muscles and the role of the physiotherapist in postpartum treatment were considered included. The excluded articles were those without specificity on the theme. Even though they addressed diastasis, they did not focus on physiotherapeutic exercises as a way to minimize the consequences on the woman's body.

Procedures

To meet the research objectives, 25 articles were selected to compose the scientific work, and only 16 were included because they met the requirements of the inclusion factors published between the period 2010 and 2017, with reference to physiotherapy in the treatment of patients with diastasis of the rectus abdominis muscle.

The scientific articles were selected according to the presentation of titles, abstracts and key words. Then, a full reading was performed as a way to identify the aspects related to the study proposal, organized the information, recorded and analyzed, according to Figure 1:

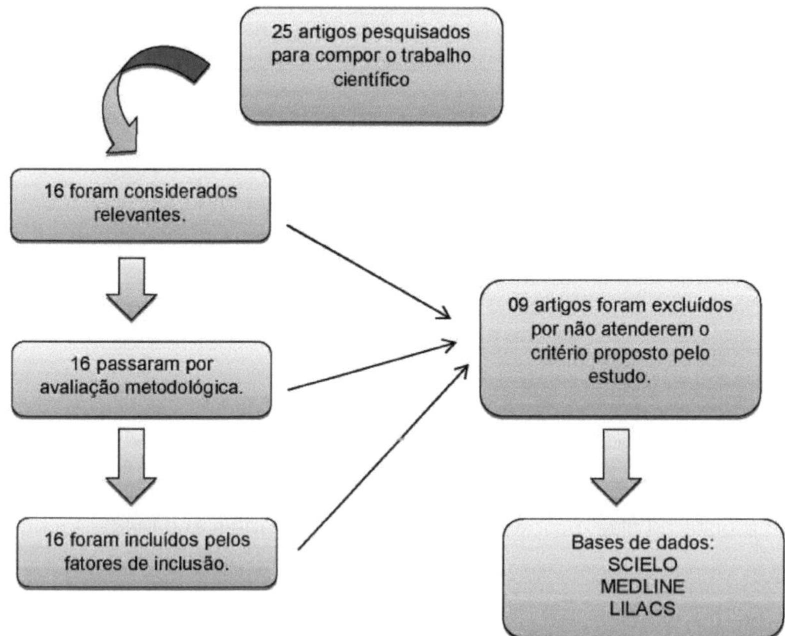

Figure 1: Scheme of organization of the researched articles.
Source: data provided by the research authors, 2017.

RESULTS AND DISCUSSION

The following descriptors were used: "delivery", "diastasis", "straight muscle", "abdominal", and "physiotherapeutic treatment". Studies were included that demonstrated the physiotherapeutic approach in women with postpartum diastasis or that contributed to the objective of this study, published between 2010 and 2017 in Portuguese.

Table 1 shows the general distribution of the articles according to the title and research base:

Table 1: Article, title and research base.

Articles	Title	Search base
N1	Physiotherapy to reduce diastasis of the rectus abdominis muscles in the postpartum period.	SCIELO
N2	Use of physiotherapeutic resources in the puerperium	MEDLINE
N3	Care of puerperal women by physiotherapy in a humanized public maternity hospital	SCIELO
N4	Diastasis of the rectus abdominis in puerperal women and its relation with variables	MEDLINE
N5	Frequency of abdominal diastasis in puerperal women	SCIELO

N6	Diastasis of the rectus abdominis muscles in the immediate puerperium of primiparous and multiparous women after vaginal delivery	LILACS
N7	Physiotherapeutic approach in rectus abdominis diastasis	SCIELO
N8	Physiotherapy in the puerperium	SCIELO
N9	Relation between physiotherapy and diastasis	LILACS
N10	The effectiveness of kinesiotherapy in reducing diastasis of the rectus abdominis muscle	SCIELO
N11	Importance of physiotherapy in the diastasis of the rectus abdominis muscles in women in the puerperium	LILACS
N12	The main physical changes in puerperae assisted in the Healthy Pregnancy Programme	SCIELO
N13	Prevalence of diastasis of the rectus abdominis muscle in puerperal women	MEDLINE
N14	Immediate puerperium care: the role of physiotherapy	SCIELO
N15	Physiotherapy intervention in diastasis of the rectus abdominis muscle (DM RA).	LILACS
N16	Physiotherapy applied to the post-natal period: diastasis	LILACS

Source: data provided by the research authors, 2017.

Among the scientific articles researched, the Scielo database corresponds to a total of 8 journals for integrative research, marking a percentage of 50% of the scenario of 16 registered files. Followed by Lilacs with 5 journals and Medline with 3, that is, 37.5%.

However, the studies that did not meet the study period and presented publications that did not deal with scientific research were eventually excluded, according to Table 2 below:

Table 2: Title, author, study, objective, sample, parameters and results.

N°	Title	Author/ Year	Study	Objective	Sample	Parameters	Results
01	Physiotherapy to reduce diastasis of the rectus abdominis muscles postpartum	MESQUIT A, Luciana Aparecida et al. RBGO Journal, v. 21, n. 5, 2010.	Longitudin al and random	To verify if physiotherap eutic intervention in the immediate puerperium can contribute to the reduction of diastasis.	50 puerperae recruited.	The control group (N = 25) underwent assessment and measurement of diastasis (6 hours and 18 hours after delivery) and the treatment group (N = 25) underwent the same assessment and	At 18 hours post-partum, the control group showed a reduction in diastasis of 5.4% and the treatment group of 12.5%, in relation to the first measurement (6 hours after birth).
						measurement above.	
02	Use of physiotherapeu tic resources in the puerperium	SANTANA, Licia Santos et al. Revista Feminina, mai, v.39, n.5, 2011.	Literature review.	To carry out a review of the non-pharmacologi cal resources available for use after childbirth in the treatment of diastasis.	Forty-three papers were selected, of which 22 were relevant to be discussed in the study.	Of the total of 22 articles, 6 related to the signs and symptoms present in the puerperium, 4 reviews and 12 on the treatment of diastasis.	The physiotherapy resources provide better adaptation of the patient after delivery and treatment of diastasis.
03	Care of puerperal women by	RETT, Mariana Tirolli et al,	Qualitative-based integrative	Contribute to physiotherap eutic	215 physiotherapy evaluation	To write the profile of puerperae	It shows that 62.3% of the puerperae

	physiotherapy in a humanized public maternity hospital	Revista Fisioterapi a e Movimento , v.12, n.6, 2012.	review.	obstetric care.	forms of puerperal women, containing demographic and clinical data, as well as specific physiotherapy records.	assisted by physiotherapy in a public maternity hospital and the care provided, aiming to contribute to physiotherapeuti c obstetric care.	presented afragma, 85.1% tympanic sound to abdominal percussion, uterine involution within normality, 87.9% pelvic floor contraction present, 30.3% edema in the lower limbs; diastasis of the rectus abdominis muscles.
04	Diastasis of the rectus abdominis in puerperal women and its relation with variables	LEITE, Ana Cristina da Nóbrega Marinho et al, Fisioterapi a e Movimento Journal > Apr/Jun; v.25, n.2, p.89-97, 2012.	Field research, using descriptive analysis and of a quantitative nature.	To compare the relationship between the value of abdominal diastasis measuremen ts and obstetric variables in puerperae.	Selected 100 puerperae.	Fertile age, in immediate puerperium.	The puerperae who presented diastasis were multiparous, multigender, aged between 19 and 30 years, having their children through normal deliveries, with short intervals between gestation periods.
05	Frequency of abdominal diastasis in puerperal women	LUNA, D. Cristina Barbosa de et al. Revista Fisioterapi a Funcional, Fortaleza, jul-dez; v.1, n.2, p. 10-17, 2012.	Frequency through cross section	To evaluate the frequency and measuremen ts of abdominal diastasis in the immediate puerperium.	89 puerperae.	Relationship between maternal weight and her BMI, hypertension and neonate weight.	Women submitted to cesarean delivery present higher values of abdominal diastasis when compared to normal delivery.
06	Diastasis of the rectus abdominis muscles in the immediate puerperium of primiparous and multiparous women after vaginal delivery	MARIANA, Tirolli Rett, et al, Revista Fisioterapi a e Movimento , v.12, n.4, 2012.	Cross-sectional observation .	To compare supra-umbilical (SU) and infra-umbilical (IU) rectus abdominis muscle diastasis (ARMD) between primiparous and multiparous women,	Included 100 primiparous women aged 21.0±4.4 years and 100 multiparous women aged 27.2±6.2 years who underwent vaginal delivery.	Data from primiparous (only one delivery) and multiparous (at least two deliveries) puerperal women who underwent vaginal delivery at least six hours after delivery.	Significant association was verified between DMRA SU and UTI and between DMRA SU, parity and age. No correlations of DMRA SU with BMI and TPP were observed, and no correlation of DMRA UI with the variables studied.
07	Physiotherape utic approach in rectus abdominis diastasis	MOURA, Lourdes Lima de; et al. Revista Fisioterapi a e Movimento , v.5, n.2, p. 12-39, 2013.	Literature review.	To analyse physiotherap y in postpartum rectus abdominis diastasis.	Public formed by women in labour and doing physiotherapy during the Nu pre natal period.	Literature review of published between 2010 and 2015.	Physiotherapy is more indicated for rectus abdominis muscle diastasis in the puerporal state.
08	Physiotherape utic actuation in the	BELEZA, Ana Carolina S. et al.	Literature review.	Describe the role of physiotherap	27 women in the puerperal period.	Data collected during 2010.	Physiotherapy is important for a better recovery

	puerperium	Hispece & Lema Journal, v.10, n.2, p. 12-27, 2013.		y in the puerperium.			of puerperae; its role consists of recovery and treatment.
09	Relationship between physiotherapy and diastasis	LIZ, Andreza Nunes de et al, Revista de Fisioterapi a e Saúde, n.27, p.9- 20, 2013.	Literature review.	To identify the main interventions during the post-partum period, including the treatment of diastasis.	36 women who make use of physiotherapy .	Women with a history of diastasis and who need physiotherapy treatment.	Physiotherapy in the puerperal period aims to promote better adaptation of the woman to the new body reality with diastasis.
10	The efficacy of kinesiotherapy in reducing diastasis of the rectus abdominis muscle	MICHELO WSK, Andréia Caroline Sampaio Alvarenga et al. Revista Brasileira de Saúde Funcional, Cachoeira-BA, v. 2 n. 2, p. 5-16, dez., 2014.	Intervenio nist, also called experiment al, random.	To verify whether physiotherap y through kinesiotra pia is effective in reducing ARMD in the puerperium	20 puerperae aged between 18 and 40 years.	Assessed and reassessed using a women's health questionnaire, 6 and 18 hours after delivery.	Physiotherapy intervention in the immediate puerperium demonstrates clinically significant reduction of ARMD in the immediate puerperium.
11	Importance of physiotherapy in the diastasis of the rectus abdominis muscles in women in the puerperium	MACCHI, Gigliola de Matos et al. Revista de Fisioterapi a e Saúde, v.5, n.9, feb./apr., p.25-37, 2014.	Literature review.	To explore the knowledge about the importance of physiotherap y in women during pregnancy and puerperium, focusing on the treatment of diastasis.	32 women Analysed during the puerperal period.	Exercises must continue during the puerperium and not only during pregnancy, thus contributing to the benefits to the body's systems, particularly the abdominal muscles.	The diastasis of the abdominal rectus muscles, although little studied, constitutes a complex and comprehensive condition, deserving attention from the professionals working in the area, especially the physiotherapy professional.
12	The main physical changes in puerperae assisted in the Healthy Pregnancy Programme	ONOFRE, Nando. Sousa; et al. Revista Brasileira de Fisioterapi a Dermato-Funcional, v.5, n.3, 2015.	Field with a quantitative, exploratory and descriptive approach.	To know the prevalence of the main physical alterations in puerperae.	25 women in the late and remote puerperal period.	In the physical evaluation the BMI was calculated and the presence of edemas, stretch marks, fibro edema geloid (FEG), melasma, diastasis of the rectus abdominis muscle (DMRA)	On the evaluation of the abdomen, flaccidity was observed in 76% of the women and ARMD in 92% of them, and in 80% of the participants the ARMD was supraumbilical .
13	Prevalence of diastasis of the rectus abdominis muscle in puerperal women	MARTINI; Elaine de et al. Revista Fisioterapi a e Movimento , v.29, n.2, Curitiba, abr./jun., 2016.	Transverse I.	To verify the prevalence of ARVD in the immediate puerperium in a sample of women assisted by the Brazilian Unified Health	88 women in the immediate puerperium	specific assessment and verified the presence of AMRD and its measurements. The measurement points were at the umbilical scar and 4.5 cm	prevalence of ARMD was 61.36%. The mean ARMD were 0.88 cm supraumbilical, 1.23 cm umbilical and 0.3 cm infraumbilical. Of the

				System and to investigate possible relations between the presence of ARVD and the number of pregnancies.		above and below it.	postpartum women who presented AMRD, 31.5% were primiparous and 68.5% were multiparous.
14	Immediate puerperium care: the role of physiotherapy	*BURTI, Juliana Schulze et al.* Journal of Medical Sciences of Sorocaba, v.3, n.9, p. 12-27, 2016.	Transverse 1.	To verify the effects of physiotherap y intervention in the treatment of diastasis in women in the immediate puerperium in a public maternity hospital in the city of São Paulo.	Fifty puerperae were evaluated, 25 vaginally delivered and 25 caesarean sections.	Diaphragmatic and abdominal re-education exercises, training of the pelvic floor musculature, metabolic exercises, manoeuvres and guidance regarding posture and treatment of rectus abdominis diastasis in the postpartum period.	The exercise protocol was shown to be effective in reducing pain and improving general wellbeing in postpartum women.
15	Physiothe rapy intervention in diastasis of the rectus abdominis muscle 1 (RADM).	VASCONC ELOS; Elias Honorato et al. Saberes Journal, v.6, jan./ago., 2017.	Experiment al and quantitativ 0.	Analyse the intervention of the physiotherapi st.	06 pregnant women aged between 23 and 31 years.	The experimental group, after the physiotherapist's interventions obtained a lower significant separation when compared to the control group.	The physiotherapist intervenes in the evaluation and treatment of the puerperal woman using resources proven through various studies to be effective in ARMD.
16	Physiotherapy applied to the post delivery period: diastasis	CORDEIRO, Mariane Alves et al, Revista Conexão Eletrônica - Three Lagoas, MG, v. 14, n. 5, 2017.	Exploratory through bibliographic al survey.	Demonstrate that physiotherap y can relieve tension, encourage muscle relaxation, strengthening , blood circulation, postural reeducation and mainly exercises to reduce diastasis.	24 pregnant women aged between 25 and 40 years.	diastasis of the rectus abdominis muscles - may initially be observed in the second trimester of pregnancy.	the help of physiotherapy can relieve tension, encourage muscle relaxation, blood circulation, postural re-education and exercises for treatment of diastasis.

Source: data provided by the research authors, 2017.

According to the highlighted Table 2, the year that showed the highest number of articles was in 2012 (04) with 25% of findings in the databases, followed by the years 2013 (03) 18.75%, 2014, 2016, 2017 (02) 12.5%, 2010 and 2011 (1) registering 6.25% of the journals.

The journal that stood out the most in its publications corresponds to the "Revista de Fisioterapia e Movimento" marking a total of 6 journals, or 37.5% of the total established for the study. While the "Revista de Fisioterapia e Saúde" presents an expected reality of 12.5% of the 16 articles organized for the study.

CONCLUDING REMARKS

The theme on the intervention of the physiotherapist in the postpartum is significant in the sense of seeking treatment for women diagnosed with diastasis. Considering that the abdominal region is seen as more requested by women in the postpartum, as well as priority areas to be treated. Being of fundamental importance to provide obstetric care, in order to cover the gravidic and puerperal period.

The theoretical references highlighted the need for evaluation of the woman by a physiotherapist after normal or cesarean delivery as a way to reduce and/or delay the appearance of rectus abdominis. Thus, physiotherapy may be performed through gentle exercises in order to strengthen the tone and increase the support functions of the abdominal muscles.

The data presented throughout the previous studies reinforced the idea that physiotherapy is more indicated with regard to diastasis in the puerperal state. This happens because of the increase in intra-abdominal pressure with the removal of the straight muscles of the abdomen. Although it has been little studied, diastasis corresponds to a complex and comprehensive condition. Thus, it deserves attention from professionals, especially the physiotherapist.

The physiotherapeutic concept indicated for the treatment of diastasis, as well as the diagnostic and therapeutic approach has been changing in recent years due to the positive results presented. The professional should act in a multiprofessional team and with an interdisciplinary approach, aiming at the completeness of the woman's assistance and avoiding future problems, such as: urinary incontinence, bad posture, low abdominal strength, etc.

Scientific knowledge about the role of physiotherapy in the diaphragmatic breathing exercise associated with the perineum, physical conditioning, relaxation, postural reeducation, strength gain of the pelvic floor muscles and abdominal muscles, is still insufficient. Needing further analysis.

The study is not restricted only to what was presented in the research, requiring further discussions on causes, consequences and treatment of diastasis. As a way to provide subsidies in terms of public health, ensure better guidance and especially treatment for women who experience the diagnosis of diastasis.

REFERENCES

ANDRADE, Michelly Fernanda Moreira de; ROCHA, Alexandra; MARTINS, Letícia. The importance of the physiotherapist performance: literature review. São Paulo, Revista Fisioterapia Brasil, v.2, n. 12, 2011.

BARACHO, Elza; Fisioterapia aplicada à obstetrícia. 4. ed. Rio de Janeiro: Guanabara Koogan, 2007, p.124-136. Revista Fisiobrasil, v.10, sep./out. 2012.

BAUER, Martin; GASKELL, George. Qualitative research: with text, image and sound. São

Paulo: Petrópolis, 2012.

BURTI, Juliana Schulze et al. Assistência ao puerpério imediato: o papel da fisioterapia. Revista de Ciências Médicas de Sorocaba, v.3, n.9, p.12-27, 2016.

BELEZA, Ana Carolina S. et al. Atuação fisioterapêutica no puerpério. Revista Hispece & Lema, v.10, n.2, p.12-27, 2013.

CORDEIRO, Mariane Alves et al. Physiotherapy applied in the postpartum: diastasis. Journal Electronic Connection - Três Lagoas, MG, v. 14, n. 5, 2017.

FONSECA, J. J. S. Metodologia da pesquisa científica. Fortaleza: UEC, 2010.

GARCIA, Maria H. M. Prado. Avaliação fisioterapêutica de puérperas. Santa Catarina: UDESC. 2007.

LAKATOS, E. M.; MARCONI, M. A. Fundamentos metodologia científica. 4.ed. São Paulo: Atlas, 2010.

LEITE, Ana Cristina da Nóbrega Marinho et al. Diastasis of the rectus abdominis in puerperae and its relationship with variables. Revista Fisioterapia e Movimento, abr/jun; v.25, n.2, p.89-97, 2012.

LIZ, Andreza Nunes de et al. Relationship between physiotherapy and diastasis.Revista de Fisioterapia e Saúde, n.27, p.9-20, 2013.

LUNA, D. Cristina Barbosa de et al. Frequency of abdominal diastasis in puerperae. Revista Fisioterapia Funcional, Fortaleza, jul-dez; v.1, n.2, p.10-17, 2012.

MACCHI, Gigliola de Matos et al. Importance of physical therapy in diastasis of the rectus abdominis muscles in women in puerperium. Revista de Fisioterapia e Saúde, v.5, n.9, fev./abr., p.25-37, 2014.

MANTLE, Jil; POLDEN, Margaret; Physical therapy in gynecology and obstetrics. São Paulo, 2010, Rev. Conexão Eletrônica, v. 14, 2017.

MARIANA, Tirolli Rett, et al. Diastasis of the rectus abdominis muscles in the immediate puerperium of primiparous and multiparous women after vaginal delivery. Revista Fisioterapia e Movimento, v.12, n.4,2012.

MARTINI; Elaine de et al. Prevalence of diastasis of the rectus abdominis muscle in puerperae. Revista Fisioterapia e Movimento, v.29, n.2, Curitiba, abr./jun., 2016.

MESQUITA, L. A. et al. Fisioterapia para redução da diástase dos músculos retos abdominais no pós-parto. Revista Brasileira de Ginecologia e Obstetrícia, v. 21, n. 5, p.267- 272, 2015.

MICHELOWSK, Andréia Caroline Sampaio Alvarenga et al. The effectiveness of kinesiotherapy in reducing diastasis of the rectus abdominis muscle. Revista Brasileira de Saúde Funcional, Cachoeira-

BA, v. 2 n. 2, p. 5-16, dez., 2014.

MOURA, Lourdes Lima de; et al. Abdominal rectus diastasis physiotherapeutic approach. Revista Fisioterapia e Movimento, v.5, n.2, p.12-39, 2013.

ONOFRE, Nando. Sousa; et al. The main physical modifications in puerperae assisted in the healthy pregnancy program. Revista Brasileira de Fisioterapia Dermato-Funcional, v.5, n.3, 2015.

RETT, M. Tirolli et al. Atendimento de puérperas pela fisioterapia em uma maternidade pública humanizada. Revista Fisioterapia e Movimento, v.12, n.6, 2012.

SCHIRMER, Janine. Assistência pré-natal: manual técnico. 3. ed., Secretaria de Políticas de Saúde - (SPS) Ministério da Saúde, Brasília: 2000, p.66-75.

SANTANA, Licia Santos et al. Use of physiotherapeutic resources in the puerperium.Revista Feminina, mai, v.39, n.5, 2011.

SILVA, A.L.C; MUNANI, D.B; LIMA, F.V; SILVA, W.O. Atividades grupais na fisioterapia: características, possibilidades e limites. Revista Rene, v.11, n. especial, 2010, p.61-71.

STEPHENSON, R. G.; O'CONNOR, L. J. Fisiologia materna. In: Fisioterapia aplicada á ginecologia e obstetrícia. 2. ed,

TALLAH A.N, TREVISANI, V.F.M. Principles for therapeutic decision making based on scientific evidence. In: Atualização terapêutica. ed. São Paulo: Artes Médicas, 2015, p.201.

VASCONCELOS; Elias Honorato et al. A intervenção fisioterapêutica na diástase do músculo recto abdominal (DMRA).Revista Saberes, v.6, jan./ago, 2017.

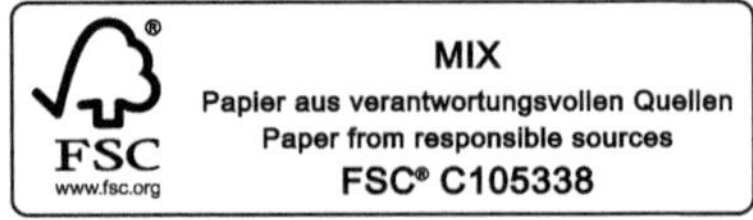

Printed by Books on Demand GmbH, Norderstedt / Germany